Alzheimer's Disease:
The Family Journey

Alzheimer's Disease: The Family Journey

WAYNE A. CARON, PH.D
JAMES J. PATTEE, M.D.
ORLO J. OTTESON, M.A.

North Ridge Press
17830 Eighth Avenue North
Plymouth, Minnesota 55447

1.888.473.5999
www.northridgepress.com

ISBN 0-9629614-2-6

Cover design by Donna Burch
Book design and production by Stanton Publication Services, Inc.,
Saint Paul, Minnesota

Contents

———

CHAPTER ONE

This chapter describes the biological, cognitive, and behavioral features of Alzheimer's disease. It identifies family care issues and dilemmas, and it introduces a phase model that can help families address care challenges.

        Phase One: the pre-diagnosis phase
        Phase Two: the diagnosis phase
        Phase Three: the role change phase
        Phase Four: the chronic care phase
        Phase Five: the shared care phase
        Phase Six: the nursing home care phase
        Phase Seven: the end-of-journey phase

CHAPTER TWO

This chapter defines the family and describes the unique features of family life. It discusses the dynamics of the family system and the need for Alzheimer's families to maintain an adaptive, learning family system.

CHAPTER THREE

This chapter describes Alzheimer's disease and defines its various stages. It discusses the nature of dementia (the "Alzheimer's world") and its effects on afflicted individuals.

CHAPTER FOUR

This chapter discusses the ways in which Alzheimer's disease constitutes a "family illness" that pervades and permeates family life. It describes some ways in which the disease invades and disorganizes family life, and it discusses some ways in which the family can meet those challenges.

CHAPTER FIVE

This chapter describes the uncertainty surrounding the pre-diagnosis phase. And it discusses some ways in which family members can move toward greater certainty—while maintaining family stability.

CHAPTER SIX

This chapter describes the diagnosis process and the family's role in that process. It discusses some ways in which family members can obtain a diagnosis and "bring it in" to family life.

CHAPTER SEVEN

This chapter describes the functional decline of the elder, and it discusses some ways in which family members can address the role changes that accompany this decline.

CHAPTER EIGHT

This chapter describes the physical, psychological, and emotional sources of caregiver strain. And it discusses some
ways in which the family can support caregivers through
maintaining the vitality of family life.

CHAPTER NINE

This chapter describes the benefits of outside help, and it discusses some ways in which the family can assess its need for outside help. It describes the process for obtaining help and for establishing a partnership with the health care system.

CHAPTER TEN

This chapter describes the benefits of nursing home care, and it discusses some ways in which family members can approach placement decisions. It defines the family's role in nursing home care, and it discusses the process for establishing a relationship with nursing home professionals.

CHAPTER ELEVEN

This chapter discusses the end of life challenges, and it describes some ways in which family members can ensure a "good death" for the elder—and find effective closure for themselves.

CHAPTER TWELVE

This chapter describes an approach to understanding behavior problems, and it discusses some strategies for relieving family frustration and turmoil. The chapter describes the differences between cognitive impairments and behavior problems. It discusses the nature and function of expectations in understanding problem behaviors. And it describes a step-by-step approach for organizing helpful responses to problem behaviors.

CHAPTER THIRTEEN

The "teaching stories" in this chapter are intended to help family members explore the material that has been discussed in the preceding chapters. The stories are intended to help family members see the ways in which various concepts apply to "real life" circumstances and problems. They are designed to help family members step back and see new options—new opportunities for addressing care challenges.

Preface

ALZHEIMER'S DISEASE POSSESSES BOTH A PUBLIC FACE and a private face. The *public* face, growing increasingly visible, troubles and disturbs us. More than four million citizens suffer from the disease—a number that is expected to double within the next twenty years. And the illness (called the "disease of the millenium") is imposing increasing burdens on family life—and on other social institutions.

The *private* face of Alzheimer's disease is seen mainly by those who live with the illness—by family caregivers and other family members who daily confront the care challenges. Families remain the major care resource for Alzheimer's victims. And they will continue to shoulder the main physical, emotional, and financial care burdens.

This book is directed toward those families. The book seeks to help families understand Alzheimer's disease as a family *illness* that affects all parts of family life. And it seeks to help families understand the illness as a family *journey* that moves through identifiable phases. These perspectives, we think, can help family members mobilize their resources and meet the care challenges as a team—dedicated to the well-being of both the patient and the family.

In the pages that follow, we will describe the family as a system—a unity of interacting personalities that possesses a boundary, a structure, and a culture. We will describe the seven phases of the Alzheimer's journey—and the major issues and dilemmas associated with each phase. And we will describe the tasks that we think can help family members move through the phases.

Our clinical experience tells us that this family systems perspective and this phase model (a kind of "road map") can help family members see more clearly the dimensions of the illness—and its impact on family life. ("What are we experiencing?" "How should we think about what we're experiencing—in each of the phases?" "How can we most effectively address the care challenges in each phase—while maintaining a vital family life?")

We recognize that various families will discover the book at various times—in various phases of the illness. Moreover, some readers will find some parts of the book more relevant than other parts—depending on the specific phase in which they find themselves. Nonetheless, we recommend that family members work through *all* the phases—from the beginning. In so doing, they will see where they've been, and they will more successfully complete later tasks—in later phases.

Acknowledgements

This book could not have been written without the contributions of the many dedicated individuals who taught us, challenged us—and inspired our thinking. Several individuals deserve special mention.

The phase model presented throughout the book was originally developed in collaboration with Irma Atkinson. Her ideas run through all our discussions, and we hope our presentation adequately reflects both the breadth of her insights and the depth of her interest in families.

We especially want to acknowledge the guidance and mentorship of Dr. Pauline Boss. Her ground-breaking work in ambiguous loss—as it applies to Alzheimer's disease—opened the door for our exploration of family emotional life, family stress, family coping responses—and other central ideas.

We wish to thank all the caring and committed colleagues who have contributed to the spirit of this book. We especially wish to acknowledge the contributions and support of Brenda Ebbitt, Joan Manthus, Marilyn Luptak, Theressa Burns, and Margaret Prodhomme.

We also wish to thank Stephen N. Barton, M.D., Ph.D., for his ongoing guidance and support.

Finally, we wish to knowledge the enormous contribution of the many families who shared their Alzheimer's journey with us. They have been superb teachers, and we hope this book successfully imparts the knowledge they've shared with us.

Wayne A. Caron, Ph.D, L.M.F.T

James J. Pattee, M.D.

Orlo J. Otteson, M.A.

Alzheimer's Disease:
The Family Journey

CHAPTER ONE

Alzheimer's Disease: Impact on Family

> *You have to begin to lose your memory,*
> *if only in bits and pieces, to realize that*
> *memory is what makes our lives. Life*
> *without memory is no life at all. . . . Our*
> *memory is our coherence, our reason, our*
> *feeling, even our action. Without it, we are*
> *nothing. . . . I can only wait for the final*
> *amnesia, the one that can erase an entire*
> *life, as it did my mother's.*
>
> — LUIS BUNUEL

THIS IS A BOOK FOR ALL THOSE WHO DAILY FACE THE Alzheimer's disease challenge—as victim, as caregiver, or as concerned loved one.

The book offers a unique perspective—a family system perspective—that rests on a fundamental premise. *The family is a system, a unity of interacting and interrelating personalities. And Alzheimer's families who develop an adaptive, learning family system will find more effective ways to mobilize their resources, to meet their care needs, and to maintain their overall well-being.*

This family systems view, grounded in the disciplines of family medicine and family therapy, is intended to help family members address the *dilemmas* that occur through all phases of the illness. These dilemmas (defined by Webster as problems with no seeming solutions) perplex and confuse. But they needn't block or inhibit effective family decision-making—or undermine family cohesion and solidarity. Properly understood, they can help family members see care issues more clearly—and address them more effectively.

Before examining some of the basic Alzheimer's care issues and dilemmas, let's look briefly at the scope and nature of Alzheimer's disease.

Alzheimer's disease: the mounting toll

Alzheimer's disease (also called *progressive dementia of the Alzheimer's type*) afflicts more than four million Americans—and imposes caregiving burdens on another twenty million family members. With no cure in sight, experts estimate that the toll will steadily mount—and that by mid-century more than fourteen million Americans will find themselves afflicted with the disease.

In recent years, medical scientists, health care policymakers, and other concerned citizens have trained increasing attention on the malady Lewis Thomas termed "the disease of the century." We're now seeing the enormous economic costs (more than $100 billion a year), and we're seeing more clearly the threats to family and social well-being.

A set of private sorrows is moving inexorably toward a true public crisis.

And, yet, the broad economic and social issues still pale next to the individual tales of loss and decline. William Shakespeare gives us this entreaty from a declining King Lear, struggling to maintain dignity and selfhood:

> *Pray, do not mock me:*
> *I am a very foolish fond old man,*
> *Fourscore and upward, not an hour more nor less;*
> *And to deal plainly,*
> *I fear I am not in my perfect mind.*
> *Methinks I should know you, and know this man;*
> *Yet I am doubtful: for I am mainly ignorant*
> *What place this is; and all the skill I have*
> *Remembers not these garments; nor I know not*
> *Where I did lodge last night. Do not laugh at me;*
> *For, as I am a man, I think this lady*
> *To be my child Cordelia.*
> *You must bear with me:*
> *Pray you now, forget and forgive: I am old and*
> *   foolish.*

The aging Lear senses his decline. And his plea for understanding and compassion, echoed throughout the centuries, evokes our sympathies. Aging exacts tolls—and old age can seem (in the words of Diogenes) like the "harbor of all ills."

We regret the infirmities imposed by age and decline. But we've learned over time to accept inevitable change. And we've learned to accommodate our aging loved ones—

while finding ways to safeguard their autonomy, dignity, and selfhood.

Although Alzheimer's disease primarily strikes the elderly, it bears little relation to normal aging losses, and it presents a far more serious picture. Alzheimer's disease— *a specific disease process*—attacks and destroys nerve cells within the brain. And, over time, the disease progressively and irreversibly changes brain structure and function.

With progressive brain cell loss, the illness eventually robs afflicted individuals of their most precious gifts: their ability to recall the past, to comprehend the present, to imagine the future—and to participate fully in family and community life.

Alzheimer's disease, a specific and identifiable illness, can be understood in terms of its *biological, cognitive,* and *behavioral* features. Let's look briefly at each.

Biological features

In 1907 Alois Alzheimer identified a disorder he called a "peculiar disease of the cerebral cortex." Since Dr. Alzheimer's early discoveries, medical scientists have continued to study the pathologies that lead to Alzheimer's disease.

In brief, we know that the disease destroys brain cells. It creates *neuritic plaques* and *neurofibrillary tangles* within the brain. And it also causes *granulovascular degeneration*—a pathology that fills the cells with fluid and granular material.

These three conditions disrupt the transmission of electrochemical signals between and among brain cells. And, with steadily increasing nerve cell loss, afflicted individuals progressively lose *cognitive* abilities—the ability to fully recall past experience and to think and reason clearly.

Thus, Alzheimer's disease can truly be seen as a specific *illness* that is characterized by a specific pattern of nerve cell death within the brain. The disease (the nerve cell loss) is progressive and irreversible—and largely untreatable.

Cognitive features

Alzheimer's disease robs individuals of their cognitive abilities—their ability to reason and to function within their environments (their "lifeworlds.") These cognitive losses occur in six general areas.

Memory
Loss of ability to recall events (recent and distant) and to identify time and place. *Example*: inability to recall names and addresses.

Language
Loss of ability to select specific words and to name objects. *Example*: inability to name parts of an object, or to follow a complex command, or to participate fully in a conversation.

Visuospatial
Loss of ability to process visual information and to recognize familiar figures and objects. *Example*: inability to correctly judge distances or to draw simple objects.

Praxis

Loss of ability to plan, organize, and complete tasks. *Example*: inability to prepare a meal or to plan a trip.

Judgment and reasoning

Loss of ability to make common-sense judgements and to formulate appropriate responses. *Example*: inability to control impulsive behaviors or to socialize effectively.

Attention and concentration

Loss of ability to maintain focus. *Example*: inability to engage in previously enjoyable activities—listening to music, reading a book, watching television.

The illness affects all six cognitive areas and imposes "global" impairment. Afflicted individuals find themselves "going backwards"—steadily losing hard won skills and abilities. And, in time, afflicted individuals lose the ability to carry out *independent activities of daily living*—telephoning, cooking, shopping, reading, writing.

As losses mount, individuals lose the ability to conduct more basic *activities of daily living*—bathing, dressing, transferring, toileting, grooming, feeding.

Eventually the progressive changes in brain structure (the increasing nerve cell loss) seriously and permanently erode the elder's ability to think and function effectively—and to behave in expected and predictable ways.

Behavioral features

Alzheimer's disease (and the resultant cognitive losses) undermine not only an individual's ability to think and reason—but also his or her ability to regulate and govern behavior. And the diminished cognitive capacity—interacting with the afflicted individual's distinct personality and social environment—lead to a set of behaviors we associate with Alzheimer's disease.

These behavioral changes occur slowly over time, and they vary among individuals. Individuals may experience mood changes. They may become depressed, sad, despairing, anxious, worried, and frightened. They may become agitated and restless—and may wander away. They may engage in seemingly purposeless repetitive activities. And they may experience thinking disturbances. They may, for example, hallucinate or develop delusions—or grow increasingly suspicious or paranoid. And they may become belligerent, aggressive, and abusive in ways that strain relationships.

These behavioral symptoms are *associated* with dementing illness—but they don't constitute the illness itself. Moreover, the elder's behaviors are influenced by various factors—personal characteristics, the social environment, relationships, and the responses of others to specific problem behaviors.

Certain behaviors may wax and wane, and individuals may find themselves experiencing "good days" and "bad days." Nonetheless, Alzheimer's disease, progressive and irreversible in nature, eventually robs afflicted loved ones of their most precious resources—their autonomy, judgment, identity, and dignity.

Memory and reasoning powers inevitably decline. Connections to self, family, and community loosen. And family members ultimately face a harsh reality. Their afflicted elder, while remaining physically and visibly present, appears to be intellectually, psychologically, and emotionally fading—like a photograph left too long in the sunlight.

For spouses and children—and perhaps for certain relatives and friends—this transformation imposes increasing challenges and duties. Caregiving needs inevitably expand and multiply—and stresses mount. And, over time, many family members also find themselves captured by the illness—victims of fatigue, frustration, and fear.

This book speaks to the millions of families who daily strive to maintain family cohesion, stability, energy, and morale in the face of difficult caregiving tasks. The book speaks to the possibilities for family change and adaptation—and to the opportunities for coming together in ways that preserve and protect (even enhance) family well-being.

Our extensive work with families has given us a sound understanding of the difficult care issues and dilemmas that surround all phases of the family Alzheimer's journey. These dilemmas (problems with no seeming solution) change over the course of the illness—as new challenges present themselves.

But we firmly believe that family members *can* understand and meet the specific dilemmas that occur in each phase of the illness. And, as they work through the specific tasks in each phase, we believe they *will* find effective ways to meet the shifting care challenges.

Let's look at some of the central Alzheimer's care issues and dilemmas.

Issue/dilemma one: Our loved one seems increasingly forgetful. Should we discuss our concerns? Or should we simply continue to "wait and watch?"

Early Alzheimer's symptoms, ambiguous and unclear in nature, can mimic certain aging signs. And family members, even health professionals, may find themselves attributing early Alzheimer's signs (mainly forgetfulness) to "normal" age-related decline—even though intellectual decline is neither a normal nor inevitable part of aging.

Moreover, many affected individuals learn to compensate for cognitive losses—they learn to conceal and disguise early decline. They may, for example, avoid activities that challenge memory and concentration abilities. And they may steer away from interactions that test their social skills. They may avoid church services, for example, or excuse themselves from participating in family gatherings, or taking shopping trips, or playing cards.

Family members also learn to compensate for their loved one's gradual losses. They quietly take over various tasks (driving and shopping) and gradually make "accommodations." These accommodations serve to maintain usual family life and to preserve established roles and relationships. But they can also disguise certain losses; and they can support and reinforce denial, minimization, and rationalization tendencies.

Thus, family members, faced with ambiguous changes in their elder's mental functioning, can find themselves asking some central questions. Are the changes we see simply signs of normal aging—or do they indicate a serious disorder? How should we express our concerns—both to our affected elder and to other family members? At what point should we "step in" and begin "taking over" certain tasks?

Uncertainty may be compounded by differences in family members' perceptions and interpretations. Various family members may see and interpret behaviors, events, and issues differently. They may develop differing views about changes in the elder, and they may form varying opinions about ways to respond.

In the face of unclear evidence, and with no clear resolution in sight, family members can find themselves confused and conflicted—unsure of what they're seeing and uncertain about how to proceed.

Issue/dilemma two: We think our loved one needs a medical evaluation. Should we seek a diagnosis now? Or should we wait for further developments?

Most families who sense (or see) a dementing disorder eventually feel a need to seek a formal medical evaluation—to obtain a diagnosis. This evaluation can provide some direct benefits. It can give family members a "fix" on reality—and can allow them to begin marshalling their coping resources and responses. An evaluation can relieve uncertainty and ambivalence. And it can help family members understand and prepare for upcoming changes in the elder.

The decision to seek a diagnosis, however, can prove difficult. It represents a major step in family life—a move into a potentially forbidding future. And many family members understandably shrink from the prospect of confronting a dementing illness—a progressive and irreversible disease that holds such large implications for family life.

Thus, the first question the family faces is *whether* to seek a diagnosis. Over time, as decline continues, the *whether* question turns into a *when* question—and ultimately into a *where* question. These perplexing questions defy easy answers, and they can lead to tension and disagreement—and even conflict.

Family members often turn initially to informal sources of information—to books or friends, for example, or to the "family medical expert." These informal information sources allow family members to "buy time"—to gain knowledge and understanding while they contemplate and deliberate the diagnosis decision.

In time, however, most families eventually require formal, professional guidance, and most seek out a professional medical evaluation.

Issue/dilemma three: Our loved one is steadily losing skills and abilities. Which activities should we limit—in order to maintain safety and well-being? And which can we preserve—in order to maintain independence and self-esteem?

Alzheimer's losses inevitably erode the elder's ability to carry out daily activities in a safe, secure fashion—even within the most familiar environments. Skills and abilities fade. And family members eventually find themselves striving to balance a loved one's safety needs against his or her freedom and self-esteem needs.

Questions about *whether* and *when* to limit an activity

can prove perplexing. A critical incident—a car accident, for example—can reveal a serious deficit and can force a needed action (the confiscation of car keys). Other less serious incidents can leave family members uncertain about whether and when, in the name of safety, to take over certain tasks and functions. ("Should we deny an activity or restrict a freedom now?" "Or should we wait—and try to maintain the usual family routines?")

Decisions to restrict a loved one's activities reverberate throughout the family system. And these "taking away" decisions (confiscating the car keys or checkbook, for example) force changes in the relationship between family members and their affected loved one.

"Stepping in" actions raise difficult questions. Who will now assist with specific tasks? "Who will begin filling the role and place of the affected elder? Who will take the lead in developing a care system?

In time, with increasing loss and decline, safety needs clearly begin to supersede autonomy and self-esteem needs. And difficult "taking away" questions begin to resolve themselves. Moreover, in time, steadily mounting care duties begin to strain family resources.

Issue/dilemma four: Our loved one requires increasing care and attention. How can we continue to provide adequate care—while protecting and fulfilling the needs, wants, wishes, and well-being of other family members?

Alzheimer's family caregivers must daily attend to elders who are steadily losing cognitive skills—who are increasingly losing memory, language, judgment, and comprehension functions.

With increasing losses, afflicted elders eventually lose their ability to understand the nature of care—and to express their appreciation. Family caregivers, burdened by increasing care duties, also find themselves frustrated by the loss of balance and "reciprocity" in the relationship.

Faced with unremitting and steadily increasing caregiving duties, family caregivers can find themselves devoting major portions of time and energy to the illness. And, in time, the family can find itself organizing around the demands of the illness—neglecting usual family routines, rituals, and activities.

Thus, family members face two sets of growing needs—those of the *elder* and those of the family *caregivers*. And all family members face two increasingly urgent questions: How can we balance our individual interests, needs, and wishes against the unceasing care demands of our loved one? And how can we continue to meet care demands—while safeguarding the overall well-being of the entire family?

Issue/dilemma five: We are exhausting family caregiving resources. Should we seek outside help? Or should we redouble our efforts and try to carry on as usual?

Steadily increasing care demands can exhaust the most resourceful family caregiving system. And most families eventually require some form of outside support (adult day care and home care, for example). Unfortunately, community dementia care resources vary widely, and family members often struggle to find needed support.

Moreover, some families find it difficult to bring needed caregiving services into their homes—and to surrender certain forms of privacy and independence. The very task of identifying and obtaining support services can become another job—a whole new set of activities that further strains an already exhausted family system.

Thus, again, family members may find themselves facing difficult questions: Do we need additional help? And, if so, what kind and how much? Where can we find needed outside help? How will we pay for it? How can we effectively integrate it into the established family caregiving system? And what are the benefits *and* burdens associated with seeking and obtaining outside care?

Issue/dilemma six: We think our loved one needs nursing home care. Should we seek such care now? Or should we wait?

Alzheimer's care demands can eventually outstrip family caregiving resources and community support services, and many families must ultimately consider nursing home care. The decision to consider or to actively seek nursing home care, however, is fraught with ambivalence and emotion— and for some understandable reasons.

First, the afflicted elder usually lacks the ability to participate in the decision—and to support the difficult transition. And many family members feel extremely uncomfortable about the prospect of placing their elder in a long-term care facility—without his or her consent and perhaps even in the face of strong objections.

Moreover, family members may disagree about the need for placement. Certain members may consider placement a sign of surrender and abandonment—a signal of disloyalty and betrayal. Feelings of guilt, anxiety, and fear can surface—leading to tension and even conflict.

In addition, family members may feel that the placement decision will limit (or close off) opportunities to maintain a supportive caregiving role. And they may find it difficult to surrender a long-established and familiar caregiving role and relationship. Co-existing illnesses in the elder and difficult medical decisions can create additional strain.

Issue/dilemma seven: Our loved one is unable to make medical decisions. Which illnesses should we treat—in order to effect cure? And which should we simply monitor—in order to maintain comfort and dignity?

Alzheimer's families frequently face difficult end-of-life treatment decisions. Dementia shortens life expectancy. But Alzheimer's patients usually die from some other disorder for which there is usually *some* available treatment (antibiotics for infections, or surgery for cancer, or medication for heart disease, or artificial feedings for malnutrition). Family members often face medical decisions that hold some possibility for prolonging life—but that offer little in the way of cure or even relief.

Without clear directives, family members can find themselves struggling to understand their options and to make the "right" decisions. And, again, they face hard questions. What decision would my loved one make in these circumstances? What are the benefits and burdens of the proposed treatment? Is the proposed treatment consistent with our elder's values—and congruent with our overall care goals?

Conclusion

The Alzheimer's family journey is marked by a series of difficult dilemmas and issues. Some kinds of dilemmas occur more frequently in the early stages; others more frequently in the middle and later stages. But all defy simple "right and wrong" judgments. And all require that family members work together as a unified and cohesive team—a coordinated system that strives to meet the elder's needs while safeguarding the family's strength, integrity, identity, and well-being.

In the chapters that follow (Chapters Two through Four), we will examine the family as a *system*. And we will discuss both the elder's experience and the family's experience with the disease. We will then describe (in Chapters Five through Eleven) the seven phases of the Alzheimer's family journey. We will discuss the two major issues associated with each phase of the journey. And we will describe the actions (tasks) that will help family members address the care challenges in each phase.

Phase One: Pre-Diagnosis Phase

Phase Two: Diagnosis Phase

Phase Three: Role Change Phase

Phase Four: Chronic Care Phase

Phase Five: Shared Care Phase

Phase Six: Nursing Home Care Phase

Phase Seven: End-Of-Journey Phase

We hope our discussion will provide a "road map" to the difficult Alzheimer's journey. And we hope it will smooth the path for Alzheimer's family members—and for all others who participate in the triumphs and sorrows of dementia care.

CHAPTER TWO

The Family and the Family System: Toward a Definition

The family: toward a definition

ALZHEIMER'S FAMILIES FACE PROGRESSIVELY DIFFICULT care issues—ongoing challenges that require continual *family system responses*. But what do we mean by a family system? And what constitutes a family system response? Indeed, what constitutes a family in contemporary American society?

Over the past decades, American family life has dramatically changed. The traditional structure (father as sole wage earner, mother as full-time homemaker, children all living under the same roof) has steadily declined—and now describes only 11 percent of all American families. Less than 30 percent of all households contain a married couple and their children.

Even in the conventional nuclear family (parents and children under one roof), large changes have occurred. More than half of wives and mothers now work. And the demands of dual careers have forced men and women to renegotiate their expectations (for themselves and for each other) and to redefine their family roles.

In the face of such diversity and shifting expectations, what then constitutes a family in early twenty-first century American society?

Definitions of *family* abound. Legal authorities emphasize binding ties of blood and marital contracts. Religious leaders emphasize the centrality of sacraments and rituals. Social scientists and psychologists emphasize emotional ties, mutual bonds of loyalty, and the family's right to define its own membership—in its own way.

Thus, a family today may possess a wide variety of members, including those connected through blood and marriage—and those who (for various reasons) simply choose to define themselves as a family.

The sociologist Ernest Burgess has given us one of the most useful definitions of a family. He calls the family a *unity of interacting personalities*. And his definition encompasses two key premises: 1) the family exists as a unity—a whole greater than the sum of its parts 2) and it exists as a set of interacting personalities—each personality no less unique for being part of a family. The family, says Burgess, is a living, changing, growing entity. And it lives as long as interaction continues to occur.

This family—this living, changing entity—strives constantly to balance its needs for both *stability* and *change*. Changing circumstances inevitably force family members to change expectations—and to redefine their roles within the family. And changes in one part of the family system lead inevitably to changes (expected and sometimes unexpected) in other parts of the system.

The family: a unique organization

A functional family possesses some unique characteristics that distinguish it from all other groups. The family group provides forms of *stability, intimacy, legitimacy, constancy,* and *diversity* that simply can't be found elsewhere. These characteristics provide large and lasting benefits to family members, and they underpin and sustain family life.

Stability

Families possess stable memberships. Kinship ties run deep, and these lifetime ties bind family members to the past, present, and future. Shared memories and experiences—and a shared family vision—lend definition and stability to family life. And lasting, lifetime relationships undergird and maintain family cohesion, solidarity, and integrity.

Intimacy

Lifelong ties also allow for special forms of intimacy and connectedness. Common histories and shared values lead to relationships that are more emotional, more personal, and more intense. Intimate family relationships lead to deep connections—and allow family members to express their real and whole selves. They allow family members to experience (in the words of T.S. Eliot) a "love that's lived in but not looked at, love within the light of which all else is seen. . . ."

Legitimacy

Society gives a special weight and legitimacy to family relationships—to relationships between husbands and wives, parents and children. Family bonds are considered sacred, and society grants a special status to family relationships and to the family group. Social institutions (the court system, for example) defer to those relationships and interfere with them only reluctantly.

Constancy

Families exist in time—they possess a past, a present, and a future. Family members are part of a long, enduring family journey—an ongoing narrative. This shared history and shared vision helps sustain the family's identity and integrity—and allows family members to transmit their values and beliefs over generations. A strong family life—a sense of togetherness—grounds family members in a set of well-understood values and expectations. And strong family relationships provide constant and enduring forms of support.

Diversity

Family life ranges across generations and life stages (up to five generations in some cases). Generational diversity—and the need to meet simultaneously the requirements of the young, middle-aged, and elderly—helps family members understand and respect differing needs and wants. Diversity strengthens family bonds and enriches and affirms the family culture. And it reminds family members that they possess a past, present, and future—and a rich store of collective wisdom.

These characteristics remind us of the invaluable (probably irreplaceable) rewards and benefits family life provides. The unique nature of family life helps family members develop strength, meaning, and purpose. And a strong, loving family life provides the commitment, comfort, and security that allow members to develop and pursue their individual goals—while calling on essential and familiar sources of support.

The family group remains always a distinct and unique organization—different in nature from any other group that we've known or ever will know. We carry rich memories and images of our families—both the family in which we were raised (the family of origin) and the family we may have created. We share unique experiences with other family members, and we retain vivid recollections of this "private world"(this family life) that only we can truly know and understand.

The family system

There is, however, another (less familiar) way of thinking about families and family life. There is a perspective that sees the family as a *system*—as a "unity of interrelating and interacting personalities" that contains a *boundary,* a *structure,* and a *culture.*

This systems view, grounded in principles of family medicine and family therapy, has been applied to a wide range of family issues. And we think it can be applied to Alzheimer's care issues in ways that enhance caregiving efforts—and promote family well-being. Let's look briefly at three basic family system concepts.

Boundary

The family system possesses a *boundary*—an imaginary line that family members draw around their family system. This boundary helps the family define its membership ("who's in and who's out"). And it marks the border between the family system and the social environment.

The family boundary changes over time, as new members enter the system (through birth, adoption, marriage) and old members leave (through illness and death). Nonetheless, most families maintain a clear boundary—a clear sense of "who's in and who's out" of the system. This boundary helps family members develop a sense of belonging, security, and connection. And it helps them identify sources of support within the family system ("Who can I turn to?" "Who can I count on?" "Who will be involved in decision-making?")

The family boundary serves critical functions. And the first step in defining the family system is to define the family boundary—to determine "who's in and who's out."

Structure

A family also possesses a *structure*—a set of "parts" that fit together in a unique way. These "parts" consist of the various family members. And the ways in which family members interact and interrelate—the ways in which their behaviors become patterned and predictable over time—determine the makeup of the structure.

This structure derives from the family's attempt to meet members' needs and to achieve family goals. And it changes over time—as membership changes (through births, marriages, and deaths) and as members' needs change.

Inevitable change forces family members to redefine their expectations (for themselves and others), and it forces revisions in behaviors and roles. Predictable and expected changes in family life (births, marriages, deaths) force changes in the family structure—in the ways family members relate and react to one another. But the family continues to function as a family. With changes, it simply revises the ways in which its members work together to meet individual and family goals.

All families face challenges—large and small. Small challenges usually require only minor changes. But larger changes can force fundamental structural changes.

Dementing illness, for example, impairs an afflicted elder's ability to carry out his or her expected role in family life. The illness—and the accompanying impairments—force other family members to adopt new roles and responsibilities. The elder's decline forces structural changes. And, in the face of mounting care demands, a family's strength (even survival) may depend on its ability to make these needed changes—to redefine expectations and to assign and accept new roles and responsibilities.

Culture

All families possess a culture—a unique set of values and beliefs that guide their choices and actions. This culture possesses its own legends and myths, its own routines and rituals, its own perceptions, its own public and private languages, its own conflict resolution methods, its own success and failure definitions, its own "language of distress," and its own explanations for illness and other misfortune.

This family culture reveals itself through the ways in which family members interact with one another—and relate to individuals and groups outside the family system. The family culture influences members' perceptions and interpretations of specific events, actions, utterances, and circumstances. It binds together disparate realities—and helps family members form a shared picture of the world. And it continually interprets behavior, explaining and "making sense" of experience—and sustaining energy, commitment, and cohesion.

The family culture remains largely covert and invisible—always present but operating in the background of family life. It is the "glue" of family life. It is rooted in deeply-imbedded core family *values*—in the enduring beliefs a family holds about itself and the world. And it powerfully influences all sectors of family life.

Values

Values underlie two central human questions: How are we to *live*? and How are we to *act*?

"How we live" values—or *end-state of existence* values—are associated with the goals of family life. ("Who are we, and what do wish to become?") And they might include ends such as freedom, security, self-respect, happiness, and wisdom.

"How we act" values—or *mode of conduct values*—are associated with behaviors and conduct. ("What actions should we choose to reach our goals?") And these values might include virtues such as honesty, ambition, competence, responsibility, and concern for others.

Individuals and families prioritize their values and order them into a value hierarchy—into a *value system*. A family's value system (its set of shared values) underlies its culture. And that enduring value system and culture shapes the family's identity and aspirations.

Even when family members disagree about specific issues (religion, politics), the family's value system continues to frame the disagreements—and to provide a common ground of understanding.

The value system (or hierarchy) usually remains sufficiently stable over time to provide a sense of continuity and meaning. But it also (ideally) maintains the flexibility to reorganize and reorder—and respond to changing circumstances.

Shared values powerfully drive family life. They undergird family culture, and they provide a sense of the family's "oughtness"—a sense of the behavior that family members *wish* to uphold and also feel *compelled* to uphold.

Values frame the goals of family life. They guide family decisions. And the ways in which the family *prioritizes* its values greatly influence its decisions—and guide its choices and actions. When faced with difficult decisions, it's useful for family members to consider both their "how to live" values—e.g., family security, freedom, happiness, self-respect, wisdom and their "how to act" values—e.g., honesty, ambition, responsibility, forgiveness, courage.

When moving toward a decision, family members will draw from specific values within each category. They will mix these values and arrange (rank or prioritize) them into a single hierarchy. The ways in which they mix and prioritize their values greatly influence their ultimate decisions. And a conscious focus on values can help family members maintain family cohesion and identity—and help them make decisions that reflect the family culture.

The challenge of change

A family, as we noted earlier, can be described as a "unity of interrelated and interacting personalities." That system possesses a boundary, a structure, and a culture. And family life is marked by regular and predictable patterns of interactions between and among family members.

The family boundary remains relatively stable over time. Various family events (births, marriages, deaths) inevitably change the nature of the boundary. But most families maintain a generally clear view of their membership ("who's in and who's out").

The family culture also remains relatively stable. The family's beliefs, values, identity, and temperament (its deeply embedded culture) holds family life together. And this enduring culture, shaped and affirmed by the family's routines, rituals, rules, and regulations changes slowly—when it changes at all.

Nonetheless, all families—like all other dynamic, living systems—face an ongoing need to change and evolve. And much of the change occurs within the family *structure*—within the family's unique set of interacting personalities.

The family deals with change (in part, at least) through altering its structure—through altering the ways in which family members interrelate and interact. Change forces new or revised expectations—and, often, new (or revised) roles.

A child, for example, grows and develops—and forces other family members to change their expectations. An elder declines—and also forces changes in expectations.

Changing family circumstances continually impel changes in family members' expectations for one another. And changing expectations impel family members to redefine their roles and relationships.

We can't avoid change—and we shouldn't. In the words of one writer, "Life is its own journey, presupposes its own change and movement, and one tries to arrest them at one's eternal peril."

Nonetheless, this need for change and adaptation must also take into account the need for stability and continuity. And a family's well-being depends in part on how well it maintains a balance between its change and stability needs.

Change and stability

Families change over time—as circumstances change and as family members are required to change the ways in which they interrelate. All families must maintain the ability to change and adapt. But families must also maintain stability—they must maintain a stable boundary, structure, and culture. Thus, all families face a central challenge: the need to maintain stability—while maintaining the capacity for growth, development, and change.

This need to maintain stability—while accommodating to change—is an ongoing challenge. In some families, the need for stability seems stronger, and change occurs only in response to pressures (sometimes taking the form of an "explosion"). In other families, change seems to occur incessantly, and these families often seem disorganized—lacking in cohesion and groundedness.

Most functional families, however, develop a balance between stability and change needs. They find ways to continually redefine roles, relationships, and expectations—and they maintain stability and balance over time.

The Alzheimer's challenge

Alzheimer's disease sternly tests a family's ability to balance its change and stability needs—and to maintain its established set of expectations, relationships, and roles (its structure).

Alzheimer's disease progressively and irreversibly steals an afflicted elder's capabilities. And the elder's decline and loss requires ongoing and continual family system change—a demand that challenges the family's ability to maintain its stability and balance and to sustain its energy and morale.

Alzheimer's families may find themselves adapting smoothly and effectively to one change—only to discover other changes moving through the system and disorganizing family life. The unrelenting care challenges can exhaust and discourage (and destabilize) any family—and for some understandable reasons.

First, the illness brings new issues and complexities into family life. Most families lack direct experience with a chronic, progressive illness—especially one (like Alzheimer's disease) that so seriously impairs mental function. And Alzheimer's family members usually find themselves sailing uncharted seas—with few guidelines to steer them through the dementia care challenges.

Moreover, the enveloping nature of the "Alzheimer's experience" changes the very nature of family life. As the elder slowly develops into an Alzheimer's patient—and other family members develop into caregivers—new tasks and expectations emerge. These new activities and responsibilities force structural changes in the family system—new and unprecedented changes in expectations, roles, and relationships.

An afflicted elder's progressive decline requires family members to gradually take over tasks and activities—and to constantly reassess and reapportion caregiving tasks. Over time, care duties intensify and multiply—and stress and strain can begin to challenge the family system at all levels.

All these factors hold the potential for seriously disrupting family balance, stability, and cohesion. Internal and external stresses can combine to paralyze coping responses and thwart planning and care activities. And many Alzheimer's families find themselves eventually organizing entirely around the illness—losing sight of the family's need for overall balance and growth.

In the face of such a daunting illness and set of formidable challenges, a family member might ask whether it's possible to maintain *any* kind of satisfying and productive family life. Can any family possibly meet the persistent and complex demands of chronic, progressive dementia?

The answer, we think, is a resounding *yes*. And the key, we think, lies in the family's willingness and ability to become an *adaptive, learning system*—a family system that anticipates and plans for change and that safeguards the well-being of all family members. Let's look more closely at this "learning system."

The adaptive, learning family system

Alzheimer's disease invades and disorganizes family life. It challenges family stability and forces family system change. This system change can occur at two levels—at the level of *accommodation* and the level of *adaptation*.

Families initially *accommodate* to encroaching illness, and family members simply increase the frequency and intensity of their usual activities ("Let's just do more of the same."). This kind of change, which theorists call "first order change," requires little or no change in family structure. And it allows families to maintain balance and to continue "business as usual."

In time, however, with the loved one's increasing losses, families must begin to *adapt*—to begin making *structural* changes. This kind of change, which theorists call "second order change," requires changes in roles, relationships, and expectations.

Accommodation, then, is a type of coping response in which family members apply the lessons of the past to new circumstances. *Adaptation*, however, is a type of coping response in which family members discard old responses and organize in new ways to meet new challenges.

Alzheimer's disease poses stern challenges—at all stages of the illness. The progressive nature of the illness, the constantly shifting care needs, continually tests and challenges family coping resources and strengths. And the ability to recognize these challenges—and to develop an adaptive "learning family system" that meets them—lies at the heart of effective family caregiving.

This book is about adaptation and about the ways in which the Alzheimer's family can meet its ongoing challenges—through all the phases of the illness. The book seeks to help the Alzheimer's family develop and maintain an *adaptive, learning system*—a self-organizing system that maintains a balance between stability and change needs and that finds ways to continually renew and revitalize itself.

In the chapters that follow, we will discuss the various phases of the Alzheimer's journey. And we will describe the various tasks that can help all family members meet the Alzheimer's care challenges. First, however, let's look at the nature of dementing illness.

CHAPTER THREE

Alzheimer's Disease: Causes and Effects

Dementia: causes and effects

ALZHEIMER'S DISEASE LAUNCHES AFFLICTED INDI-viduals on a difficult and arduous journey. To understand the nature of this journey, one first needs to understand the nature of dementia—its causes and effects.

Dementia commonly refers to the development of cognitive deficits that lead to decline in mental function—to decline, for example, in memory, language, judgement, concentration, praxis (ability to organize and complete tasks), and visuospatial function (ability to organize objects and to orient one's self).

Dementia may derive from a number of conditions, some of which (in rare cases) are reversible. Most dementia, however, derives from either Alzheimer's disease or multiple infarcts (small strokes that occur over time)—or a combination of the two.

These two conditions account for more than ninety percent of dementia cases—but their effects differ. An infarct (a stroke) is more likely to cause a focal deficit—an impairment in a specific part of the brain. And these focal impairments may remain chronic and stable over a period of time—or may, in time, even improve.

Delirium, another disturbance in consciousness, sometimes resembles dementia—but it derives from different sources. An illness (congestive heart failure) or an infection (pneumonia)—or certain toxins or medications—may induce delirium. Withdrawal from certain drugs (alcohol) and medications (benzodiazapine) can also induce delirium.

Delirium often eludes ready diagnosis. But when the underlying cause is discovered and treated, the delirium usually fades, and the patient usually recovers.

These focal impairments and deliriums pose problems. But their effects pale in comparison to the effects of *progressive dementia-Alzheimer's type*—a specific disease that gradually destroys nerve cells within the brain and that eventually affects all parts of the brain. The effects of Alzheimer's disease, progressive and irreversible, lead inevitably to cognitive impairment, functional decline, and behavioral change. And they slowly erode an afflicted individual's ability to function in his or her "life world."

Let's look more closely at the nature of this global decline in brain function—and at the specific cognitive, functional, and behavioral changes that occur over time.

Cognitive impairment

Alzheimer's disease changes brain structure and chemistry in ways that lead to cognitive impairment—to the loss of intellectual and mental abilities. As we noted in Chapter One, these cognitive impairments occur in six domains:

Memory

Afflicted individuals initially encounter memory difficulties. They grow increasingly absentminded and forgetful, and they lose ability to learn new material—and to remember previously learned material. In advanced stages, they may lose the ability to identify family members—or even to remember their own names.

Language

Afflicted individuals lose language skills. Initially, they may encounter difficulty in choosing words. In time, they begin to rely on fewer and fewer words. Their conversation becomes increasingly vague and empty. And they eventually lose full ability to use written and spoken language.

Praxis

Afflicted individuals lose the ability to plan, initiate, and conduct tasks. They may engage in needless, repetitive activities. And they may lose the ability to make simple and familiar gestures—and to use familiar implements and tools.

Visuospatial

Afflicted individuals lose the ability to orient themselves within their physical environment. They may wander and become lost. They lose the ability to fully interpret visual stimuli—to recognize and identify familiar faces and objects. They may, for example, lose the ability to correctly draw the face of a clock—and then place the hands at a specific time.

Judgement and reasoning

Afflicted individuals lose judgment and reasoning skills. They may act impulsively and take risks (driving risks, for example). They may make unrealistic assessments of their abilities—and engage in unusual and inappropriate behavior.

Attention and concentration

Afflicted individuals lose the ability to maintain focus and concentration and to sustain purposeful, long-term activity. They may lose sight of a task's purpose—or become easily distracted, especially in busy social settings.

Certain impairments—impairment in memory, for example—exhibit themselves more obviously than others. And certain symptoms show up more quickly in some patients than in others. Afflicted elders will exhibit various patterns of impairment. But in time, with increasing nerve cell loss, they will all experience impairment in all areas of cognitive functioning.

Functional impairment

Cognitive loss leads ultimately to functional impairment—to increasing loss in the ability to carry out fundamental daily living tasks. These tasks divide into two broad categories: the more complex *instrumental activities of daily living*—the IADLs—and and the more basic *activities of daily living*—the ADLs.

Cognitive losses steadily erode overall function, but the functional losses show up first in the more complex instrumental activities (the IADLs)—housework, for example, or the tasks associated with shopping, cooking, and financial management.

With increasing nerve cell loss, Alzheimer's individuals gradually lose the ability to carry out the more basic activities of daily living (the ADLs)—bathing, dressing, feeding, transfer (moving), and toileting. They may become incontinent and lose bowel and bladder control.

Each activity can be assessed in terms of three standards: 1) the ability to perform independently, 2) the ability to perform semi-independently, and 3) the inability to perform. An assessment of these functional abilities—both the IADLs and ADLs—can help family members measure losses and determine existing function. An assessment can help families match care services to needs—and initiate more focused interventions.

Behavioral change

Cognitive losses lead also to unpredictable and troubling behaviors—and to seeming changes in personality. Amiable and energetic individuals may become demanding and list-less. Afflicted elders may become passive, apathetic, rest-less, irritable, angry, and depressed. They may gradually become less sensitive to social cues—and less capable of meeting social expectations. Their social relationships may change, and the very nature of their personality may seem to change.

Many afflicted elders simply exhibit exaggerated versions of long-held traits and characteristics. Stubborn individuals may grow more stubborn. Anxious individuals may grow more anxious. And lovable individuals may even grow more lovable.

Many unusual and unpredictable behaviors are simply responses to stimuli that the elder cannot fully understand and interpret. An unexpected tap on the shoulder, for example, might be interpreted as a threatening gesture. Or an unexpected noise or a simple reflection in a mirror might be interpreted as an intrusion—and might startle and unsettle the elder. The inability to correctly perceive and interpret events in the environment can create suspicion, paranoia, fear and distrust—and can foster other unwanted feelings and states of mind.

Behavior problems hold the potential for seriously disrupting and disturbing family life. They may derive from dementia, but they may also be rooted in other conditions and illnesses. And family members should consult a physician before drawing conclusions about the sources of functional decline and behavior changes.

The progressive stages of Alzheimer's disease

Cognitive and functional loss is progressive, and decline moves through predictable stages. Various researchers have developed various descriptions of these stages. We think the Barry Reisberg model for the Stages of Alzheimer's Disease provides an especially good "road map" to the afflicted loved one's journey through the disease stages. A slightly modified version of his scale is shown below.

Stage 1: no cognitive decline (normal).

• No complaints and no evidence of memory deficit.

Stage 2: very mild cognitive decline (forgetfulness).

• Some complaints of memory deficits (losing objects, forgetting names).

Stage 3: mild cognitive decline (early confusional).

• Early clear cut deficits:
    a) difficulty traveling to a new location
    b) difficulty maintaining work performance standards
    c) difficulty choosing words and recalling familiar names
    d) difficulty retaining written material
    e) difficulty remembering new names
    f) difficulty keeping track of valuable objects

Stage 4: moderate cognitive decline (late confusional).

- Clear cut deficits:
    a) difficulty recalling parts of personal history
    b) difficulty maintaining concentration
    c) difficulty traveling, handling finances, etc.

Stage 5: moderately severe decline (early dementia).

- Signs of early dementia:
    a) increasing need for help with basic activities
    b) inability to recall important aspects of current life—e.g., address, telephone number, names of certain family members (grandchildren), names of schools attended
    c) difficulty identifying time and place
    d) difficulty retaining basic knowledge of selves and others (spouse's name and names of children)
    e) difficulty dressing appropriately.

Stage 6: severe cognitive decline (middle dementia).

- Signs of middle dementia
    a) difficulty remembering name of spouse
    b) difficulty remembering recent events
    c) difficulty remembering past experiences
    d) difficulty identifying surroundings
    e) difficulty traveling to familiar locations

    f) difficulty maintaining regular sleep patterns
    g) delusional behavior (speaking to imaginary figures)
    h) personality and emotional changes
    i) anxiety symptoms
    j) inability to determine a purposeful course of action.

Stage 7: very severe cognitive decline (late dementia).

- Signs of late dementia
    a) may lose all verbal ability—and frequently all speech
    b) may require assistance with all activities of daily living (bathing, dressing, toileting, transfer, continence, and feeding)
    c) may lose basic psychomotor skills (ability to walk and move)

These stages represent the major steps in the afflicted elder's journey. Each individual moves through the stages in his or her own unique way, and no individual moves neatly from one stage to the next. Moreover, not all individuals exhibit the same losses to the same degree—within the same stage. Nonetheless all afflicted individuals eventually move through all the stages.

The Alzheimer's world

Reisberg's stages provide a kind of "road map" to the ways in which Alzheimer's disease progressively disables an afflicted individual. But the stages represent only one part of the Alzheimer's journey. Alzheimer's individuals also find themselves moving through another kind of journey—through a psychological, emotional, and spiritual pilgrimage that can't be defined in terms of disease symptoms and stages.

Alzheimer's disease moves the elder into a different world. And, over the years, we've tended to assume that the elder moves silently (even painlessly) into this world—staying generally unaware his or her transformations and losses.

We now know, however, that afflicted individuals (at least in the early and middle stages) often stay painfully aware of their losses. They understand the progressive nature of the illness and the ways in which they are steadily losing skills and abilities. And they strive mightily to compensate for loss and decline—and to maintain a place in family life.

These heroic efforts deserve our admiration. And we can only wonder at the afflicted elder's emotional, psychological, and spiritual experience. But when we begin to see not only the nature of the Alzheimer's losses but also the nature of the afflicted loved one's experience, we gain glimmers of the Alzheimer's journey. When we begin to recognize the ways in which the elder's world is *diverging* from the "normal" world, we begin to deepen our understanding of the Alzheimer's experience—and the family's experience.

Diverging worlds

Global mental decline, decline in all areas of cognitive function, robs individuals of a precious and irreplaceable resource—their memory and their ability to access the past. With progressive cognitive loss, individuals over time lose the ability to reflect on their life experience—to understand it, to appreciate it, and to draw from it.

Cognitive loss (especially memory loss) moves afflicted individuals into an increasingly narrow world in which memory grows increasingly spotty and unreliable. Short-term memory may falter, and individuals may lose the ability to recall recent events and experiences—while retaining vivid memories of certain distant events.

Moreover, an afflicted individual's memory may skip randomly across a lifetime of experience. And this inability to see one's past in terms of a continuous, uninterrupted narrative can move individuals toward a "here and now" world—toward a contracted world that seems somehow more comprehensible.

Afflicted individuals lose a sense of continuity. They lose the ability to integrate the past with the present—and to imagine a future. Their life "story" becomes disjointed, and they begin to lose their "map"—their ability to "connect the dots." Without a clear memory of the past, they find it difficult to keep themselves "fixed" in the world. They find themselves increasingly unable to reach into the past and to draw from a gathered pool of experience and wisdom.

This kind of disorientation—this inability to fully recall a past and to fully imagine a future—interferes with the ability to "make sense" of the present. And, with an increasingly jumbled past and unfathomable future, afflicted elders become increasingly focused on their immediate experience—on their "here and now" reality.

Robbed of the ability to reflect on the past, to understand the present, and to contemplate the future, the elder is increasingly forced into the present—into an increasingly narrow scope of human experience.

For unimpaired family members, the afflicted loved one's world seems increasingly foreign and unfathomable. And for the afflicted loved one, the ordinary world—the world of his or her family members—seems increasingly incomprehensible and "jumbled."

The reality of each world seems out of rhythm (out of "sync") with the other. And both the afflicted elder and his or her nonafflicted family members find themselves struggling to connect their worlds—to bridge over into one another's reality.

The elder's move into an increasingly constricted, "here and now" world cannot be halted. But when family members see their relationship to the elder in terms of diverging worlds and a progressive "mismatch"—when they begin to understand the gap between "two worlds"—we think they take a long step toward developing more empathic and effective responses. And we think they may develop more effective responses to problem behaviors.

They may, for example, abandon futile attempts to pull the afflicted loved one back to "ordinary" reality. They may learn to validate their loved one's reality, and they may see more clearly that the elder's behaviors (in many cases, at least) are simply attempts to create or maintain a more comprehensible (albeit narrower) world.

For many family members, the gap between the two worlds (the world of the afflicted and nonafflicted) may seem small and manageable in the early stages. But over time, with progressive loss, family members may feel that they're losing (or have lost) their connections to their elder.

Nonetheless, family members who learn to enter into their loved one's "contracted" (and contracting) world may make interesting discoveries. They may find that parts of their emotional relationship have remained alive and vital—and that they can connect at the nonverbal level (through touch, gesture, and facial expression, for example). And they may find that the impaired family member has re-tained the capacity to experience joy and happiness—and to maintain a place in family life.

Alzheimer's disease launches two journeys—the indi-vidual's biological, emotional, psychological, and spiritual journey and the family's psychosocial journey (its experi-ence with the illness).

Each journey possesses a special and distinct charac-ter—and each defies pat solutions and "one size fits all" ap-proaches. But when we see the family experience in terms of two journeys, we see more clearly the ways in which Alz-heimer's disease evolves into a "family illness." And we see more clearly the need for an adaptive, learning family sys-tem that continually accommodates and adapts to shifting realities and care challenges.

Let's look more closely at the family experience.

CHAPTER FOUR

Alzheimer's Disease: A Family Illness

Alzheimer's disease: the family experience

IN THE PRECEDING CHAPTERS, WE BRIEFLY OUTLINED the dilemmas Alzheimer's families face in various phases of the Alzheimer's journey. We described some ways in which the family can be understood as a system—as an identifiable entity that possesses a boundary, structure, and culture. And we examined the specific nature of Alzheimer's disease—its origins and its effect on afflicted individuals.

In this chapter, we will focus on Alzheimer's disease as a "family illness"—as an "invader" that disrupts and "disorganizes" long-established family routines, rituals, rules, roles, and relationships. And we will explore the nature of the *adaptive, learning family system*—its uses and its relation to Alzheimer's care issues.

Let's first consider Alzheimer's disease as a family "invader."

Alzheimer's disease as invader

Alzheimer's disease strikes at family life through the cognitive impairments it creates in the elder. Cognitive losses rob afflicted individuals not only of hard-won skills—but also of the qualities that make them unique and special.

Over time, with steady loss and decline, the elder begins to seem "there" but "not there"—physically present but increasingly psychologically and emotionally absent. Family members mourn the losses. And they find themselves struggling to understand and accept the cognitive and behavior changes—and to maintain their emotional connections with their loved one.

In time, increasingly unpredictable behaviors begin to stand between the elder and his or her family members. The illness—an uninvited, unwelcome intruder—begins to insidiously and relentlessly invade all domains of family life. It takes up residence. It begins to dominate family routines and rituals. And, for many families, the disease becomes a "family illness"—an enveloping, pervasive, inescapable presence that casts a dark shadow over all family activities.

Alzheimer's disease as disorganizer

Alzheimer's disease not only invades the family domain—it *disorganizes* family life. It alters roles and relationships. And it disrupts the family's stability—the family's need to maintain an established *boundary,* a cohesive *structure,* and an enduring *culture.* Let's briefly examine each in relation to the *invading* and *disorganizing* nature of Alzheimer's disease.

Boundary

Alzheimer's disease raises two family boundary issues. First, the illness places increasing care demands on the family. And these mounting care duties eventually require a collective family response. In order to organize a family response, family members must first determine who's in and who's out of the family *system*—and then determine who's in and who's out of the family *dialogue*.

Answers to these questions will determine (in part at least) who will participate in decision-making activities and who will ultimately enter into family caregiving activities.

Family members must also make ongoing decisions about the ways in which the elder will participate in normal family activities. In the early and (perhaps) middle stages of the disease, the elder's participation in family routines, celebrations, and rituals can be useful and welcome. In later stages, involvement can unsettle the elder and disrupt family life—and, consequently, rob all family members of needed enjoyments and satisfactions.

Thus, family members must constantly examine boundary issues. Who's in? Who's out? To what *extent* is an individual family member in or out? To what extent should we (and can we) include the elder in family activities?

Answers to these questions help family members clarify (and keep clarifying) the family boundary. Dialogue and discussion around boundary issues will help family members organize a collective response to care challenges—and will help them keep the family organized and focused.

Structure

The invasive and disorganizing nature of Alzheimer's disease also raises critical *structure* issues. First, as the elder's cognitive losses mount, family members find themselves changing their expectations for their loved one—and, consequently, changing the nature of a long-standing and treasured relationship.

Again, difficult questions arise. What can I expect of my afflicted loved one—now and down the line? What does he or she expect of me? How can I best meet my elder's expectations—while meeting my own obligations and responsibilities?

Second, mounting caregiving duties force changes in expectations among nonafflicted family members. And, since a collective family response is inextricably linked to *expectations*, more difficult questions arise. Who's capable of doing what? Who's willing to do what? What general forms of support can we expect? What specific forms of support can we expect from specific individuals—within specific disease stages?

Certain family members may be willing and able to participate in one way, at one disease stage—and another way (or no way) at another disease stage. Or they may need to adjust their participation as the disease progresses. Thus, changing realities and care demands require an ongoing "expectations" dialogue—an ongoing family conversation that focuses on changing roles and relationships.

Expectations define roles, and they define the tasks that family members are willing and able (and expected) to perform. When family members agree on specific tasks (on who will do what and when), the family structure tends to stay organized. When they're unable to clearly define expectations, the family structure (its set of roles and relationships) tends to become disorganized.

Thus, family members must constantly consider the family system's structure. They must continually consider the expectations they hold for themselves (as individuals) and for one another. Are the caregiving tasks clear and appropriate? Are they realistic? Can the caregivers perform them? Are expectations clear? Do they need to be changed and revised? When and how?

Answers to these questions will help the family stay organized. Clear expectations and well-defined roles will help the family maintain stability in the face of a disorganizing and destabilizing illness that permeates family life and challenges family resources.

Culture

Alzheimer's disease creates dilemmas—problems with no seeming solution. And, in the face of dilemmas, family members often develop differing perceptions and judgements. These differences can lead to tension, disagreement, and conflict—and can seriously disorganize family life.

Families with clear and well-defined values and beliefs can more easily resolve vexing dilemmas. Family members who reflect on their family values—and who make decisions that are congruent with their family culture—will more readily resolve value conflicts. And they will make decisions they can more easily "live with." ("To what extent should we preserve our elder's freedom?" "To what extent should we preserve and protect his or her safety?" "What's constitutes a good balance?")

Maintaining stability in the face of change

As we noted in Chapter Two, all families face change and transformation. And any change (expected and unexpected) disorganizes family life—to some degree. Most families adapt to regular change and maintain a stable family organization. They adapt and move on.

Alzheimer's disease, however, poses some special challenges. Its dementing and progressive nature strikes at the heart of the family's ability to stay organized. And the *uncertainty* surrounding the illness—together with its *enveloping* nature—holds the potential for *demoralizing* and *deenergizing* family life. Let's look at each of these disorganizing features—one at a time.

Ambiguity

Alzheimer's disease, insidious and progressive in nature, introduces uncertainty into family life. This ambiguity (difficulty in knowing) is related to some basic questions about the illness. Is it real? Will it get worse? If so, to what extent and at what rate? How should we respond—now and down the line? What does the future hold—for the elder and for the family?

Alzheimer's families strive for greater certainty. They seek a "roadmap" that will guide them through difficult terrain and help them resolve perplexing dilemmas. This quest is understandable. But, unfortunately, the illness defies "cookbook," "one-size-fits-all" approaches. Each afflicted individual's experience with the disease is unique, and each family's approach is unique—shaped by its own unique temperament, identity, and set of resources.

Moreover, Alzheimer's disease resembles few other illnesses. Most families possess little or no experience with a dementing illness. And this lack of experience—together with a lack of clear care guidelines—fuels ambiguity (difficulty in knowing) and creates ambivalence (difficulty in deciding).

Ambivalence

The Alzheimer's journey is marked by ambivalence and by a series of dilemmas—problems with no seeming solution. Family members constantly face unpalatable options. And again and again they find themselves in a state of ambivalence—a state that can express itself in two ways: 1) family members may be unable to determine "right" courses of action (we don't know) or 2) they may not like any of their options (we see the choices—we just don't like them).

With no seemingly good alternatives, families find it difficult to mark their successes. With no clear successes, family members can develop a sense of failure and futility—a sense that they're unable to make any effective decisions. ("What difference will it make?")

Enveloping and pervasive nature of the illness

Alzheimer's disease seeps into all sectors of family life. And, over time, it can envelop and permeate family routines, rituals, rules, and relationships. The illness enters into every family interaction and casts a shadow over almost every family activity. The relentless monitoring and care demands can, in time, "engulf" individual caregivers—and can ultimately "take over" family life in ways that undermine individual and family well-being.

Demoralizing and deenergizing nature of the illness

Alzheimer's disease brings sadness and grief into family life. The progressive nature of the illness and the chronic feelings of grief can steal opportunities for hope and joy—and force families to reassess their hopes and expectations. The illness can erode the family vision and undermine the "family dream." And it can ultimately degrade hope and optimism—and finally demoralize the family system. In the face of a gloomy and forbidding future, the family can get stuck in the "here and now"—moving from one crisis to another without plan or purpose.

The Alzheimer's challenges, with their constant demands on family strength and resources, require the family to continually and continuously identify and nurture its strengths. But these strengths are considerable—and they are enduring.

They include the ability to maintain a sense of connection and belonging (helped by a clear boundary), the ability to communicate and solve problems (helped by a clear structure and set of expectations), and the ability to maintain a sense of commitment to common goals (helped by clear values and a clear culture).

A family's response to the Alzheimer's "invader" is also powerfully shaped by its *temperament* and *identity*.

Family resources for meeting the challenges

Temperament

Family temperament consists of the characteristic activity patterns and response styles that families exhibit—as they go about shaping their daily routines and resolving their problems. Family temperament is also shaped by the ways in which various family members interact and "fit together."

Family temperament is the product of three fundamental properties: 1) the family's typical energy level, 2) the family's preferred interactional distance, and 3) the family's characteristic behavioral range.

The family's *energy level* refers to its behavioral activity. We describe some families as high-energy ("hot") and some as low-energy ("cool"). The family energy level is affected by the intensity of interactions within the family—by the activity level of family members and by the passion that pervades family life.

The family's preferred *interactional distance* refers to the degree of involvement between and among family members. Some families are "close"—family members spend time together and know a great deal about one another's lives. Other families are less close—family members maintain a looser connection with one another.

The family's *behavioral range* refers to the family's flexibility and creativity. Some families value new experiences and creative approaches. Others prefer consistency, stability, and predictability.

Different combinations of these three dimensions produce vastly different family temperaments. There are no right and wrong temperaments. But some understanding of temperament can help the Alzheimer's family recognize its behavioral traits and perhaps respond more effectively to care challenges.

Family identity

Family *identity* can be viewed as a set of shared values, beliefs, and attitudes that give the family its unique nature—and that distinguish it from other families. This shared belief system—this set of family paradigms, themes, myths, and rules—strongly shapes a family's view of reality. And it influences the family's sense of "who we are" and "how we go about our business."

The family identity rests on certain beliefs about membership (who's in and who's out) and on certain long-held values. It rests also on recollections of the family history—on recollections of past shared experiences. And memories of past illnesses and past caregiving experiences—recollections of the ways in which the family met previous challenges—can help the family shape effective approaches to Alzheimer's care demands.

Family identity plays powerful role in transmitting

shared beliefs across generations. The ability of the family to maintain its core identity determines whether the family will take on *dynastic* qualities—whether it will transmit its traditions and beliefs across generations.

Illness—especially a chronic, progressive, dementing illness like Alzheimer's disease—can seriously erode family identity. And it can seriously undermine family routines, family rituals, and short-term family problem-solving activities. Each of these three observable behaviors—routines, rituals, and problem-solving activities—provides a window into the nature of underlying family regulatory processes. And each deserves brief mention.

Routines, rituals, and problem-solving activities

Family identity is constantly affirmed through daily *routines*, family *rituals*, and *short-term problem-solving activities*.

Routines

Routines consist of the background behaviors that give structure and form to daily life—and that impose some order on the pace and patterning of daily activities. Daily activities—meal preparation, housekeeping, shopping—add structure and predictability to daily family life. These daily routines lack flash, and, to the outside observer, they often look repetitive and boring. But they convey a sense of order and comfort—and they strongly reflect a family's temperament.

Rituals

Rituals consist of special behaviors that possess a strong symbolic content. Family celebrations (Christmas, Passover, weddings, baptisms) call forth highly cherished behaviors. Family traditions (birthdays, vacations, reunions) hold special meaning for family members. And patterned routines (dinnertime, bedtime, leisuretime rituals) are imbued with a sense of specialness.

Rituals affirm and transmit family values and culture, and they help preserve the constancy of the family's internal environment. Rituals celebrate a common identity and build family morale. They affirm the family's roots and maintain the family's connection to the larger community. And they reinforce the loyalty of the participants—while sustaining and nourishing family life.

Short-term problem-solving activities

Short-term problem-solving, the third category of observable regulatory behaviors, is the one most closely linked to family stability. Families strive to balance stability and change needs. And they maintain balance and constancy by responding to the challenges that threaten stability— and by developing and activating the discrete and focused problem-solving behaviors that help them meet specific challenges. Once met, the problem-solving behaviors usually recede into the background.

Chronic illness can disturb all these family regulatory behaviors. Alzheimer's disease can begin to shape family identity. Family members can begin organizing around the illness, and the illness can become the organizing principle for all kinds of family behavior. The disease can *invade* family routines and rituals—and can severely challenge family problem-solving abilities and activities. Ultimately, the illness can disrupt and disorganize family temperament and identity—two essential family strengths.

Conclusion

In face of all these challenges, family members might ask, "Is there any good reason to think that we can effectively address this disease—that we can cope with an illness that holds such large potential for permeating, enveloping, deenergizing, and demoralizing family life?"

We think the answer is an emphatic *yes*. And we think the key lies in the ability of the family to develop an adaptive, learning system that meets the care challenges—while maintaining overall family well-being through all its various phases.

Just as we can describe the afflicted individual's journey in terms of a series of *stages*—so too can we describe the family's experience in terms of a series of *phases*. Each family will experience the illness in its own unique way. But each family, throughout the course of its journey, will face certain common issues and tasks.

In the upcoming chapters, we will discuss the seven specific phases that constitute the Alzheimer's family journey. And we will describe the specific tasks within each phase that we think will help families meet care challenges—as they develop and maintain an adaptive, learning family system.

Some understanding of these phases, we think, will allow family members to develop a "roadmap"—a guide to where they've been, where they're at, and, perhaps, where they're going. The map, we hope, will allow family members to lift their gaze—to understand the order in which specific challenges arise and to see a path through the difficult terrain.

Some families, at the point they pick up this book (this "map"), will have passed through one or more of the phases. But we think these families can benefit from working through early tasks—in earlier phases. In so doing, they will see where they've been, and they will more successfully complete later tasks—in later phases.

CHAPTER FIVE

Phase One:
The Prediagnosis Phase

PHASE ONE, THE PREDIAGNOSIS PHASE, IS MARKED BY family uncertainty and ambivalence. The slow onset of Alzheimer's disease—and its insidious entry into family life—raises difficult questions.

Are certain worrisome behaviors (forgetfulness and memory loss, for example) signs of aging—or early signs of a dementing illness? Should we be concerned? Or should we leave well enough alone—for now? Should we discuss our concerns with other family members? And, if so, with whom? Should we discuss our concerns with our "affected" loved one? And, if so, when—and how?

Uncertainty pervades the prediagnosis phase, and many families, in Phase One, find themselves "in limbo"—increasingly worried about changes in their loved one's behavior and function but uncertain of their source.

Family uncertainty, in Phase One, is fueled by *ambiguity* (difficulty in "knowing") and *ambivalence* (difficulty in "deciding"). And ongoing uncertainty holds the potential for undermining family coping efforts and disorganizing family life.

Families can't perfectly resolve all the Phase One uncertainty issues. But some understanding of their sources can help family members relieve strain and stress—and reduce the potential for disagreement and conflict.

Let's look at two basic Phase One issues.

Issue one: ambiguity—difficulty in knowing

Early Alzheimer's disease, with its subtle symptoms and slow, silent onset, defies attempts to "name" and "label." In the face of puzzling behaviors, family members face tough questions. Is it real? Is it changing? What are we seeing? Uncertainty pervades the Phase One family experience, and it derives from some specific sources.

Insidious onset

Unlike Parkinson's patients (who may develop tremors) or multiple sclerosis patients (who may lose strength), early Alzheimer's patients show few obvious symptoms. Early losses, expressing themselves mainly in forgetfulness, may mimic "normal" aging signs—and may raise little concern. ("Dad's just having a "senior moment.") And family members, in Phase One, may find it difficult to discern a "real" disorder.

Inconsistent expression of illness

Many early Alzheimer's signs and symptoms express themselves in somewhat erratic and inconsistent ways. That is, they may come and go, wax and wane. Affected individuals may experience "good days" and "bad days"—days when they seem forgetful and confused and days when they seem relatively normal and untroubled.

Fatigue, pain, infection, medications, sleeplessness, and exciting or tiring events (a family celebration, for example) may temporarily draw out certain symptoms. Then, following a period of rest—or after some form of treatment—the symptoms may recede.

Moreover, early Alzheimer's symptoms often mimic symptoms of other disorders that also cause individuals to withdraw and to tire easily (urinary tract infection, for example, or arthritis, or influenza). And the lack of clear, concrete, specific symptoms—together with the potential for "good days" and "bad days"—can cloud the family's attempts to see an emerging pattern and picture.

Ability to accommodate

Uncertainty derives also from the remarkable ability of all family members, including the elder, to accommodate—to compensate for loss and decline.

Affected elders learn to "pass." They may, for example, begin to avoid social circumstances that challenge their abilities—and reveal their losses. Or they may angrily dismiss questions about certain troubling behaviors. Or they may simply ignore the questions. These accommodation strategies blur evidence of dysfunction, and they further fuel uncertainty and apprehension.

In addition, family members, in Phase One, may begin to "take over" small tasks and to assist in small ways. ("Why don't you let me drive, Dad. My car is right out in front.") These helpful responses ease certain difficulties, but they also may serve to mask a loved one's losses—and to further extend the period of uncertainty.

Differing perceptions and interpretations

Family members may develop differing views about troubling behaviors. They may interpret signs and symptoms, incidents and events, differently. And these differing perceptions and interpretations can thwart the family's attempts to define a problem and to reach a consensus.

Moreover, an affected elder's behavior may vary from time to time and place to place—and this, too, can affect family members' perceptions. One family member, for example, may see the elder only at certain times and in certain places—and may, consequently, form one set of conclusions. Other family members, especially those who regularly see the elder (perhaps daily), may form different conclusions. And all these differing views and perceptions (and conclusions) can further complicate the family's attempt to develop a clear picture and a firm consensus.

Lack of clear guidelines

We look to our health care system for answers—for definite and clear diagnoses. We strive for medical certainty, and we seek assurances that our concerns are being fully addressed. And, yet, to this day, some illnesses (like Alzheimer's disease) continue to defy easy and ready diagnoses. What, for example, constitutes "normal" memory loss? What degree of forgetfulness indicates dementing illness? Which specific behaviors point toward Alzheimer's disease?

The subtle and inconsistent expression of early Alzheimer's symptoms—together with differences in elders' abilities and previous levels of function—defy attempts to develop "one size fits all" diagnostic guidelines.

Thus, in the early stage of the disease, physicians and other health care professionals—and family members—may find themselves in a "watch and wait" period. Professionals, in Phase One, may need time to ascertain a pattern of loss. And family members may need more time to monitor behavior and to gather additional information.

Issue two: ambivalence—difficulty in deciding

Ambiguity (difficulty in knowing) fuels uncertainty. Is it real? Is it changing? Is it serious? And uncertainty fuels ambivalence (difficulty in deciding). Again, difficult questions arise. Should we discuss our concerns? And, if so, with whom? Should we seek help? And, if so, to whom should we turn?

For some families, the course of action may seem unclear. For other families, the course of action may seem clear—but all the options may seem unattractive (even repellant). In both cases, a family may experience ambivalence and may encounter both difficulty in deciding and difficulty in making concrete decisions. Other factors can also contribute to ambivalence and uncertainty.

High stakes

Alzheimer's disease poses grave threats to family life. And the high stakes—the potential threats to family well-being—can block or impede important family discussions and decisions. Family members understandably shrink from the prospect of confronting a progressive, irreversible, incurable disease. The stakes are high—and the potential implications for family life severe. These high stakes can lead to denial and minimization. They can cause family members to delay action—to wait and "see what tomorrow brings."

Fear of conflict

Ambivalence (difficulty in deciding) is also frequently rooted in a fear of conflict. Differing perceptions and observations can lead to differing interpretations—and to disagreements about courses of action. The desire to avoid conflict and to maintain family peace and stability is understandable. But excessive fear of conflict can inhibit dialogue and discussion—and can stall needed decision-making and problem-solving activities.

Disagreement and fear of conflict can also lead family members to begin solving problems "on their own"—without benefit of family consultations. These well-intentioned individual actions derive from understandable desires to "fix" problems—to take action. But individual efforts can undermine a coordinated family system response and erode a team approach to issues and problems.

Stigma

In a society that highly values intellectual abilities and economic productivity, the threat of dementing illness (and the illness itself) repels many citizens. And the stigma associated with dementia (in all its forms) can block family discussion and action.

In his eighteenth-century novel, *Gulliver's Travels*, Jonathan Swift described the demented "struldbrugs" as people with "no remembrance of anything but what they learned and observed in their youth and middle age, and even that . . . imperfect." These fictional characters were, said Swift, "despised and hated by all sorts of people."

Three centuries later, many Americans continue to shun and stigmatize (even ridicule) demented individuals. And family members, sensitive to this social stigma, are understandably reluctant to place a "demented" label on a beloved family member. Without clear evidence of illness, family members may avoid difficult discussions and decisions—and, again, extend the period of uncertainty.

Helplessness

Finally, in the face of potential Alzheimer's disease, family members may develop a sense of helplessness. They may see few options, and they may seemingly throw up their hands. ("Why talk about Mom's poor memory—what good will it do?" "Why open this can of worms—what will it accomplish?") These feelings of helplessness—rooted in fear and a seeming lack of viable options—may further fuel ambivalence and uncertainty.

Uncertainty pervades the Phase One family experience. And uncertainty can hobble (even cripple) the family's ability to cope with an elder's increasing loss and decline. Uncertainty, however, needn't overpower or undermine family decision-making. When family members understand its causes—when they understand that their feelings derive from specific and understandable sources—we think they can move forward with greater clarity and consensus.

The following tasks will help family members cope with uncertainty and move more easily through the difficult and perplexing Phase One period.

Task one: observe and record signs of illness

The family's ability to paint a picture—and to develop consensus—rests heavily on its ability to observe and record the elder's behavior. Each family member will observe and record in his or her own special way. But a few general guidelines can help all family members develop shared perceptions and understandings.

Look for general signs of decline

Impairment is ultimately "global" in nature. That is, it reaches into all six cognitive domains—memory, concentration, judgment, language, orientation, and task completion. And it ultimately impairs abilities in all domains.

In the early stages, however, signs and symptoms may show up more clearly in one domain than in another. And early losses (in most cases) initially affect the ability to carry our complex tasks. Moreover, as we've noted, certain symptoms may wax and wane—may come and go. And certain "environmental" factors (the social setting, for example) can draw out certain symptoms.

In addition, decline and loss must be measured against previous level of function—against the range of previously demonstrated abilities. These previous levels of function can vary widely among individuals. Some memory loss in an absent-minded individual, for example, might raise little concern; memory loss in an elder with a demonstrated "photographic" recall might raise more concern. Individuals who perform highly precise work (engineers and accountants, for example) may exhibit losses in clearer and more obvious ways.

Thus, family members, in Phase One, should look for decline in *overall* function—in the ability to perform a range of basic and interrelated tasks (driving, socializing, recalling names, managing finances, preparing meals). Family observers should look for overall decline and for *patterns* of decline. They should look for specific "incidents"— departures from expected and established behaviors.

And, when examining and discussing incidents, their dialogue will benefit from a focus on the facts, on the four *Ws*—"Who," "What," "When," and "Where." Who were the actors involved in the incident? What was the setting? When and where did the incident or event occur? A series of incidents may reveal a pattern (a pattern of forgetfulness, for example), and several patterns may develop into a picture.

If, indeed, an elder is afflicted with Alzheimer's disease, the illness (progressive and irreversible in nature) will inevitably reveal itself. An elder, for example, may initially show signs of mild forgetfulness. But, in time, the elder will inevitably exhibit decline in several domains of cognitive function. Incidents will grow more frequent and serious. Patterns will emerge. And a picture will inevitably emerge.

Family members (observers all) might wish to keep a diary or a journal—a record of specific incidents (who, what, when, where). Periodic review of written records can help the family identify worsening patterns and see a developing picture.

Family members may also find it helpful to record the *intensity* of their emotional reaction to an incident—the degree to which a specific behavior distressed them. These records can help family members reach consensus. And, during the diagnosis phase, they can prove invaluable to both family members and medical professionals.

Avoid speculation

In Phase One—the "watch and wait" phase—family members should strive to avoid the "whys" of specific behaviors and incidents. "Why" questions lead to unproductive speculation. And speculation steers individuals away from "here and now" issues and concerns. Early speculation about causes can interfere with observation and reporting tasks—and can stall consensus building activities. Family members will benefit, in Phase One, from avoiding the "whys" and staying with the observable facts. This approach will help the family assemble a more accurate picture—and perhaps a stronger consensus.

Task two: communicate through dialogue

Effective communication strategies will help all family members work through the critical Phase One period. And the concept of *dialogue*, we think, can help family members address early uncertainty and ambivalence issues. But what exactly is dialogue? And how does it work?

Dialogue

Dialogue (as we use the term here) consists of a *conversation*—a nonjudgmental exchange that allows all family members to freely explore and share their observations and feelings. Dialogue seeks to help individuals think together—to collectively analyze an issue and to develop a picture.

Open and nonjudgmental dialogue allows family members to express differing observations, perspectives, and feelings in an atmosphere of tolerance and acceptance. It aims at the *sharing* of information ("What are we seeing?") and the *expression* of feelings ("I'm worried, and sometimes I feel sad.").

As family members add new observations, perceptions, and feelings to the old, themes emerge and deeper understandings develop. Family members move toward consensus and desired courses of action—and toward a communication stage we call *discussion.*

Discussion

Discussion differs from dialogue in one major way. Dialogue seeks to help individuals exchange information and share feelings. Discussion seeks to help individuals move toward concrete decision-making and problem-solving activities.

In discussion, individuals focus on the information they've acquired—and then begin identifying priorities, exploring options, and laying out acceptable courses of actions ("What *should* we do?" "What *can* we do?")

Effective *discussion* grows out of free and open *dialogue*. Each form of communication serves a distinct purpose. Dialogue seeks only to help individuals freely express themselves in a nonjudgmental setting. Discussion seeks to help individuals make decisions and solve problems.

These two forms of communication set the foundation for a systems approach to complex dilemmas. And we think both forms foster an "adaptive, learning family system" that strives always for consensus and effective action.

Family members often wonder whether to include their "affected" elder in early conversations. The question eludes easy answers (and we'll take it up again in later chapters). But generally, we think some form of the Golden Rule applies. Exclusion can lead to secrets, and secrets can stifle dialogue and discussion—and can foster suspicion and distrust. Each family will handle the "inclusion issue" in its own way. But inclusion, in Phase One, allows the elder to enter the dialogue and to help with early planning and problem-solving efforts.

Task three: mobilize the family system

Family members, in Phase One, sense (but can't confirm) the presence of an "intruder"—an "invader" who seems bent on disrupting established family routines. This invader—this set of problematic behaviors in the elder—can disorganize the family system and undermine family function.

Thus, as family members continue to observe and record, dialogue and discuss, they must also attend to the *integrity* of the family organization. They must attend, that is, to the *family system*—its boundary, structure, and culture. And they must strive always to maintain the family's emotional, psychological, and spiritual resources.

Let's look at some boundary, structure, and culture issues—as they relate to Phase One issues.

Boundary

As we noted in Chapter Two, The family boundary consists of the line that family members draw around their family system. This boundary helps family members determine "who's in and who's out" of the system? And it helps them address important questions. Who's involved? Who's contributing? Who's available? Who's relating to family concerns?

Under normal circumstances, the family boundary stays relatively stable and clear, and family members usually find little reason to examine and clarify it. But changes in an elder's behavior and function bring special stresses and challenges into family life. Monitoring and observation needs increase, and care needs begin to develop. ("Who's going to help Dad drive?" "Who's going to help with the shopping?" "Who's going to pay the bills—and balance the checkbook?")

As needs increase—and as family members find themselves increasingly "stepping in"—the need to define the family boundary takes on greater importance. ("Who's available?" "Who's willing and able to help?" "Who can we count on—and for what?")

So, even in Phase One, before confirmation of any dementing illness, family members will benefit from assessing the family boundary (who's in and who's out) and identifying expectations (who's prepared to do what—and when). Answers to these questions will help lay the foundation for the development of a family caregiving system—if, indeed, the family eventually finds that Alzheimer's disease has invaded family life.

Structure

As we noted earlier, each family system possesses a structure—a familiar and predictable pattern of interactions that occur between and among family members. This structure—the set of expectations that shape roles and relationships—develops slowly over time. And, over time, these predictable interaction patterns help the family maintain stability, cohesion, and solidarity.

Under normal circumstances, the family structure (like the family boundary) stays relatively stable. Family members interact in accustomed and predictable ways. And they learn (ideally at least) to negotiate changes or differences in expectations.

These expectations may change little during the Phase One period—as family members continue their "watch and wait" activities. But if decline and loss continue—and if diagnosis proves that Alzheimer's disease has indeed entered family life—family members will inevitably find themselves redefining expectations and assuming new roles.

The Alzheimer's "invader" (a family "disorganizer") will inevitably force structural change—changes in expectations and consequent changes in roles and relationships. And family members who focus on family structure issues in the Phase One period will better equip themselves to address upcoming care issues—if, as we've said, Alzheimer's disease has truly invaded family life.

Culture

A family's culture—its set of shared values—powerfully affects its approach to the Phase One dilemmas. Values guide choice and action. They shape the family's identity and vision. And they strongly influence family decision-making activities.

Values provide the "glue" that holds family life together. And a family's values—its commitment to certain goals and behaviors—guide and shape its approach to change and illness issues. (Who are we? What are our goals? What are the means we choose to attain them? What do we wish to become?)

In the face of troubling changes—in the face of a yet unnamed "invader"—an early and consistent focus on values can help family members establish goals and can lay a foundation for later decision-making. Early and ongoing reflection on family goals and values can help the family maintain its identity and integrity. And it can help family members maintain the customs, beliefs, routines, and rituals that both support and reflect the family culture.

Task four: accommodate and maintain family stability

Family members who suspect a dementing illness face a special challenge. They must accommodate to their affected loved one's increasingly unpredictable behavior—while continuing their "watch and wait" activities and maintaining (to the extent possible) family life "as usual." They must learn when to *accommodate*—and when to *adapt*. And they must learn to establish not only the means for change—but also the means for maintaining stability and the status quo.

Family members *accommodate* and *adapt* constantly to changes in family life. Accommodation and adaptation are ongoing features of "normal" family life—necessary adjustments that are driven by specific and anticipated family events (births, deaths, marriages, the natural development of children, and the natural and expected changes in elders).

Accomodation

Accommodation occurs when one family member simply helps another family member fulfill his or her family role. Accommodation is aimed at maintaining family life "as usual"—and it occurs continually.

In the course of ordinary family life, family members *accommodate* to change through increasing the frequency and intensity of their activities—while maintaining their usual roles, functions, and tasks. Accomodation activities don't require large changes in expectations or major transformations in roles and relationships. That is, they don't require adaptations.

Adaptation

Certain events and changes in family life, however, do require *adaptation* responses—changes in expectations and consequent changes in roles and relationships. Certain developments within family life (births, deaths, marriages, illnesses, the natural maturation of a child, the expected decline of an elder) force changes in expectations. And these changed expectations force family *adaptation*.

With adaptation, one family member begins to perform another family member's role (rather than simply helping fulfill the role). And one or more members move into a new set of expectations and a new (or at least revised) role.

Adaptations and accommodations occur at various levels in family life, and they're "triggered" by events within and outside the family system. A family might decide, for example, that an elder can continue to maintain his or her finances—but that a family member will assist in balancing the checkbook or paying the bills. This is an *accommodation*. Family members at some point, however, may decide to confiscate the checkbook and take control of finances. This is an *adaptation*. The family is now fulfilling a role—and not simply assisting the elder in fulfilling a role.

Accommodation helps families maintain stability in the face of early change. Accommodations (changes in frequency, intensity, and quantity of assistance) do not require system *adaptation*. Rather, they serve to maintain family stability and established family life through an uncertain period of change. ("I'll help you drive Dad." "Let me help you pay the bills.")

Accommodation, a set of specific responses to changing circumstances, allows family members to maintain usual family life—while continuing their monitoring and recording activities. Accommodation allows the family to "buy time" while it moves toward greater certainty—toward an understanding that a real illness has invaded family life. Accommodation allows family members to maintain "life as usual" while they ponder the possibility that life as usual may not go on—and that, indeed, major changes may be imminent.

In time, with the loved one's increasing loss and decline, accommodation and early adaptation strategies may no longer meet changing conditions and circumstances. Family members may feel compelled to seek answers and to "name" an increasingly apparent disorder. And they may reach consensus that a medical evaluation is required. But where does one begin? And to whom does one turn?

CHAPTER SIX

Phase Two: The Diagnosis Phase

PHASE TWO, THE DIAGNOSIS PHASE, IS MARKED BY A series of difficult questions. Should we seek a diagnosis? If so, should we seek it now—or should we wait? To whom should we turn? What is our role in the diagnostic process? If Alzheimer's disease is confirmed, how do we handle ("take in") the reality of the illness?

The decision to seek a diagnosis represents a major step in family life—a move into an uncertain and potentially stressful future. And family members may (understandably) shrink from the prospect of confronting a dementing illness—especially one that holds such potential for transforming family life.

Nonetheless, in time, the need to "name" an increasingly apparent problem eventually impels most families to seek medical advice. And we think that families who understand diagnosis as a *process* (a series of steps) and as a *collaboration* (between family members and health professionals) will move more easily through the diagnosis phase.

Issue one: diagnosis as process

The diagnosis process begins within the family, and it begins with two questions: Why should we seek a diagnosis? and When should we seek a diagnosis?

Why seek a diagnosis

Medical evaluation provides some real benefits. Some families learn, for example, that the elder's thinking and memory impairments are related to a treatable medical condition (severe depression, reaction to a medication or alcohol, irregular heartbeat that can lead to strokes). And, with this knowledge, family members can move quickly to resolve (or at least relieve) the memory problems.

For most families, however, evaluation usually confirms a long-standing suspicion: the elder has been stricken by a progressive, dementing illness (probably Alzheimer's disease) that is steadily eroding cognitive skills and slowly undermining basic abilities.

This information—shocking, painful, and disturbing—can arouse the family's deepest fears. But it can also prove helpful. A diagnosis can help "clear the air." It can provide reassuring knowledge that baffling behaviors are related to a specific medical condition—to an *illness* that can be understood and addressed. It can help family members move from ambiguity to certainty—from ambivalence and indecision to action. And it can help the family envision a future that includes the Alzheimer's disease reality.

When to seek a diagnosis

The decision to seek a diagnosis may be "triggered" by accumulated strain—and by increasing difficulty in accommodating to the loved one's mounting losses. The decision may also be triggered by a "critical incident"—by a major event (an auto accident) or perhaps by a series of less serious events (bouncing yet another check).

These "trigger" events create strain, and they often add to a growing climate of strain. Moreover, they contribute to a sense of urgency—a sense that the family must begin to define the problem and identify the needed courses of action.

But even in the face of crisis, family members may find themselves disagreeing about the need for a diagnosis. And the objections to a medical evaluation are understandable. ("How can we get Mom to see a doctor?" "We're overreacting to normal aging signs." "This will only create more difficulties.") Disagreement can add to family strain. And strain can lead to the kind of conflict that impedes calm and effective decision-making.

Thus, the question of *when* is closely related to the issue of family strain. Ambivalence and indecision can foster strain, and accumulated strain can begin to impair family interactions. When strain begins to adversely affect family life—and when care demands begin to outstrip accommodation strategies—the family system begins to seek answers. The system that has thus far managed uncertainty begins to seek greater clarity—and some assistance in "naming" an increasingly obvious disorder.

Families differ in their ability to tolerate strain, and elders differ in the ways they exhibit impairment. And it's difficult to define a precise point at which a family should seek medical evaluation.

In general, we think families should seek help when communications between family members begin to break down—and when strain begins to disrupt family relationships and family life.

With good dialogue and open communication, most families in time reach a consensus that it's time to relieve uncertainty—that it's time to seek a medical diagnosis.

Issue two: diagnosis as collaboration

Diagnosis can be viewed not only as a process that occurs over time—but also as a collaboration between and among family members and between the family team and the health care team.

Dialogue helps family members share their perceptions, observations, and feelings—and helps them develop shared meanings and understandings. ("What are we seeing?" "What are we feeling?" "How should we proceed?") Dialogue helps family members find areas of agreement—an important first step in reaching consensus and developing a team approach.

This team approach can foster effective forms of collaboration with the health care system. Both the family system and the health care system bring unique forms of knowledge and expertise to the diagnosis process. And both systems benefit from a collaborative relationship. Strong collaboration helps family members and health care professionals develop clear understandings and expectations. And it helps them find effective ways for identifying and using community health care resources.

Again (as in Phase One) many family members wonder whether to include the elder in Phase Two family discussions. And, again, the question defies easy answers. Opinions vary, and even medical professionals disagree. Some professionals think inclusion unnecessarily taxes an affected individual. Others believe that inclusion benefits all family members—including the elder.

Our experience tells us that most affected elders (in the early stages) understand their difficulties. They handle difficult information with surprising strength and fortitude. And attempts to shield a loved one from difficult truths can undermine trust and foster suspicion.

Thus, we think that all family members—including the elder—should be included in Phase Two family discussions. Full inclusion fosters collaboration and cooperation throughout the family system, and it protects the family from the corrosive effects of secrecy and deception.

The following tasks describe ways in which the family can effectively obtain a diagnosis and effectively "bring it into" family life.

Task one: obtaining the diagnosis

After working through the *why* and *when* questions, most families initiate an approach to the health care system— and continue their search for answers.

Various kinds of health care professionals are equipped to assess cognitive impairment—and to conduct physical, neurological, mental status, and psychiatric examinations. In our view, however, a primary care physician is especially well-suited to conduct an initial Alzheimer's disease evaluation.

These physicians focus on the "whole person." They are able to assess the combination of physical ailments that might be causing memory problems. And they are equipped to evaluate an individual's overall physical and psychological health.

Moreover, primary care physicians possess a knowledge of community health care resources—and an overview of the health care system. They can refer patients to other specialists and services, and they can guide family members through the community health care system, They are also prepared to address a range of medical conditions (infections, heart disease, and hypertension, for example) that can occur in any stage of the disease. And they are equipped to provide medical counsel and support through all phases of the Alzheimer's journey.

A primary care physician might choose to conduct the entire evaluation within his or her clinic. Or the physician might refer the family to another specialist—one who specializes in dementia diagnosis and care. Many dementia clinics offer education, support, and research programs that provide special benefits to families.

A physician's success in developing a clear picture depends greatly on how clearly the signs and symptoms of cognitive impairment reveal themselves, how clearly the course of symptoms can be established (stable, worsening, or improving), and how well the physician can rule out other contributing disorders (medication reactions, emotional disturbances, heart problems).

In many cases, the dementia symptoms are obvious, and the loved one's pattern of decline clearly indicates the presence of Alzheimer's disease.

Often, however, the examining physician requires additional information. And both the physician and the family members may need to temporize—to "buy time" and continue their "watch and wait" activities. This need to temporize and to continue gathering information can prove frustrating. But for many families it's the only course available.

Health care professionals constantly remind us of the need to seek professional medical advice at the first sign of trouble. Early Alzheimer's disease, however, often defies certain and absolute diagnosis. And early diagnosis of Alzheimer's disease, although helpful, does not strongly enter into the prevention of life-threatening conditions.

Thus, the need to temporize (to "buy time") will not necessarily threaten the immediate health of an elder. Neither will the use of "high tech" diagnostic tools necessarily hasten diagnostic certainty. Alzheimer's disease, progressive in nature, always (eventually) reveals itself. But many families—even after the initial medical evaluation—must continue their "watch and wait" activities.

The need to maintain a "holding pattern," however, needn't halt the family's active participation in the diagnosis process. Family members can continue to gather and record and share information, to assess and analyze it—and to continue their partnership with the health care professionals.

This partnership is a critical part of the diagnostic process. Physicians require family input. And a firm partnership helps the family develop an active role—it helps both family members and health professionals achieve their objectives.

Having obtained the diagnosis, the family must now bring the illness into family life. And family members must work through the three tasks associated with psychologically and emotionally assimilating the illness.

This assimilation (this "taking in") process occurs in three ways—in three steps. First, family members must develop an understanding of the diagnosis ("What is it?"). Second, they must develop ways to acknowledge, accept, and express their feelings about the diagnosis. ("How is it affecting us emotionally and psychologically?") And, third, they must develop responses to the demands of the illness. ("How can we most effectively address the illness? What changes do we need to make—as individuals and as a family?")

Task two: understanding the diagnosis

More than fifty-five illnesses, some nonprogressive, can cause dementia. But the disorder regarded as "dementia of the Alzheimer's type" shares essential characteristics: 1) it derives from brain damage and brain cell death, 2) it is progressive, and 3) it is incurable.

These disease characteristics present family members with a set of challenging (sometimes overwhelming) realities. And family members face a critical challenge at this point. They must find ways to develop a collective response to the illness, and they must come together as a team. At the point of diagnosis, family members must find ways to stay connected—a critical element in the family's efforts to support one another and to begin assimilating the diagnosis.

Family members first need to ensure that they understand the information the physician (or other health professional) has conveyed to them. They can test their comprehension of that information by restating the information to themselves—or to one another. This restatement exercise may reveal gaps in understanding and may help family members formulate and address important questions.

What is the progression of the disease? How can other illnesses contribute to decline in function? Is the illness a genetic disorder—and are other family members at risk? What are the community services that can help ease caregiving burdens and maintain the elder's quality of life?

These kinds of questions help family members identify knowledge gaps. They orient the family toward needed courses of action. And they help family members develop shared understandings about the nature of the disease—its meaning and its implications for family life.

Task three: accepting the diagnosis

Once family members have "taken in" the diagnosis at the *thinking* (or understanding) level, they must then "process" the diagnosis at the *feeling* level. Diagnosis shocks the family system—and there's little that can blunt that shock. All family members will benefit, however, from dialogue that allows them to both understand the diagnosis and to *emotionally accept it.*

Certain feelings inevitably arise—grief, sadness, fear, apprehension. Some family members may find themselves expressing anger. Others may find themselves withdrawing and distancing themselves from family life. Regardless of the initial response to diagnosis, it's critical that all family members find ways to confront and "process" their emotional responses to the event. And, again, dialogue can help.

Family dialogue helps family members share their feelings about the diagnosis and helps them find ways to process their emotions together—as a family. Dialogue helps family members articulate, express, and *share* their feelings.

Dialogue—open communication that does not attempt to resolve issues—allows family members to express their feelings and share their feelings and understandings about the disease. It relieves feelings of aloneness and isolation. And it helps move the family toward a major and necessary conclusion. *We are now a family that is coping with Alzheimer's disease. We must now orient and adapt to this new reality. And we must organize to meet the new challenges.*

Families who are unable (or unwilling) to "take in" the diagnosis—at both the understanding and feeling level—face some specific hazards. The inability to understand and accept the diagnosis can foster an *under-response* or an *over-response.*

The under-response—the inability to understand and accept the information—may resemble *denial.* The *over-response*—the view that the diagnosis represents a catastrophe—may resemble *panic.* And family members who "catastrophize" the experience may find themselves burdened with fear and despair and troubled by erratic behavior.

Both extreme reactions can occur within the same family, and both seem to arise when family members are unable to freely express and resolve their feelings. Both reactions can seriously undermine problem-solving and coping activities. And both can interfere with the family's need to emotionally assimilate the diagnosis and to begin operating as a team.

Task four: acknowledging reality of the illness

Alzheimer's disease "invades" family life, and, left unchecked, it will eventually occupy all the "rooms" in the family home. Thus, in addition to understanding and accepting the diagnosis, family members must find ways to take charge of the illness—to "stay on top of it."

But take charge of what? Medical options are few. Although certain medications may relieve certain symptoms, the disease remains largely untreatable. And family members, in Phase Two, often find themselves struggling to formulate care approaches—and to meet new challenges.

We think that families at this early post-diagnosis point can take one major action. *They can fully acknowledge the reality of the illness, and they can fully bring it into family life.*

This acceptance does not require the family to organize all its activities around the illness. Indeed, such a focus can unnecessarily disrupt family life. It does, however, position family members to take action—to take charge of the illness. And family members will benefit, in Phase Two, by asking three central questions. What parts of family life has the disease taken over? What parts does it threaten? And what parts can be preserved? Answers to these questions will help guide initial decisions and actions—and will help all family members move forward.

Again, we think family members should share diagnosis information with the elder. Secrets seem to inevitably impair family communication, and secret-keeping can ultimately create more distress than the temporary discomfort that may accompany clear, open, direct communication.

For the Alzheimer's family, early post-diagnosis day-to-day life may change little. But the ways in which family members think about themselves and their afflicted elder—and about their futures—will inevitably change. With diagnosis, the afflicted elder has become a patient with an identifiable disease. And family members must begin to think anew—and to see themselves as a family with an Alzheimer's illness.

Thus, acceptance involves not only intellectual understanding and emotional "taking in"—it also involves the development of a new family identity. The evidence that the family has intellectually and emotionally processed the new reality—and has accepted its new identity—lies, we think, in its *willingness and ability to announce the presence of the disease.*

Many families are reluctant to share the diagnosis with friends and associates. They may fear the stigma attached to dementing illness, and they may wish to shield the loved one. We've found, however, that the family's willingness to share the diagnosis—to "go public" with friends and associates—helps make the diagnosis even more "real." Disclosure helps family members avoid denial reactions and other unproductive responses. And it opens up opportunities for others to provide support and guidance.

Moreover, the "public" announcement is sometimes the first concrete post-diagnosis step the family takes together—as a team. And this exercise in teamwork can set the stage for other collective decisions and actions.

The following note from President Ronald Reagan, written to the American public shortly after his diagnosis, eloquently and gracefully acknowledges the presence of Alzheimer's disease.

RONALD REAGAN
Nov. 5, 1994

My Fellow Americans,
I have recently been told that I am one of the millions of Americans who will be afflicted with Alzheimer's Disease.

Upon learning this news, Nancy & I had to decide whether as private citizens we would keep this a private matter or whether we would make this news known in a public way.

In the past Nancy suffered from breast cancer and I had my cancer surgeries. We found through our open disclosure we were able to raise public awareness. We were happy that as a result many more people underwent testing. They were tested in early stages and able to return to normal, healthy lives.

So now, we feel it is important to share it with you. In

opening our hearts, we hope this might promote greater awareness of this condition. Perhaps it will encourage a clearer understanding of the individuals and families who are affected by it.

CHAPTER SEVEN

Phase Three:
The Role Change Phase

PHASE THREE, THE ROLE CHANGE PHASE, IS MARKED by an inescapable reality: a treasured loved one is losing the ability to carry out independent, adult activities (driving, shopping, managing finances). And family members, in Phase Three, must now find ways to meet emerging care challenges—while maintaining family stability and well-being.

With increasing loss and decline, the afflicted elder, in Phase Three, is becoming a *care receiver*—and family members are becoming *caregivers*. The family that has accommodated to loss and decline through the Prediagnosis and Diagnosis phases must now, in the Role Change phase, begin to adapt—to reorganize in ways that foster new relationships and address mounting care challenges.

Issue one: the changing scene

Increasing cognitive loss—and consequent loss of function—lead inevitably to increasing dependence. And the family, in Phase Three, faces a time of transition, a period in which family members must address not only emerging care issues but also changes within the family system—changes in expectations, roles, and relationships.

The elder's increasing decline—his or her inability to fully carry out everyday activities—requires family members, in Phase Three, to begin "stepping in" and assisting with specific tasks. These "stepping in" actions force changes in family members' relationship with the elder. And, in this transitional period (this "sorting out" period), family members find themselves "betwixt and between"—uncertain about when and how to "step in" on specific activities and unsure about their relationship to an increasingly dependent loved one.

These early stepping in actions hold broad implications for family life. They change the expectations family members hold for the elder, and they change expectations family members hold for themselves. And all these changed expectations—driven by the stepping in actions—inevitably alter family roles and relationships.

Stepping in actions mark a major step in the family journey. For the elder, they represent a loss of freedom and autonomy. For the family, they represent the beginning of family adaptation—the beginning of changes in the family structure (in roles and relationships) that will occur through all phases of the Alzheimer's journey.

But these necessary interventions can prove difficult. Elders value their long-held roles and their places in family, and they're reluctant to relinquish them. Family members respect these roles, and they, too, are reluctant to begin "taking over." They struggle to accept the structural changes (the changes in roles and relationships) that accompany changes in the elder's abilities. And they find themselves dealing with feelings of grief and sadness—with a sense that life has irrevocably changed and will continue to change.

Thus, the family's first challenge is to understand the ways in which the stepping in actions are changing expectations—and, consequently, transforming roles and relationships.

The second challenge is to understand the ways in which early stepping in actions constitute the beginning of a family caregiving system—the first step in a family adaptation process that will continue throughout the entire Alzheimer's journey.

Issue two: the emerging caregiving system

The family, in Phase Three, faces critical questions. What kind of help does our elder need? Who is able to help—and how? Who is willing to help—and when? In answering these questions family members begin to develop caregiving roles. And in fulfilling these roles, family members begin to develop a caregiving system.

Through the specific interventions that occur over time, family members begin to change their expectations (for themselves and for the elder)—and they gradually change their roles. Family routines, rituals, and rules—and the organization of day-to-day family life—begins to change. *And all these changes, in our view, constitute the essence of family adaptation and reorganization.*

With the development of a distinct caregiving system,

the family, in Phase Three, is undergoing a major transformation. Family members are organizing themselves in new ways—and becoming more closely involved in day-to-day care activities. Just as the arrival of a new baby forces family members to assume new roles and responsibilities, so too does the elder's increasing dependency force family members to assume new tasks and responsibilities—and to begin working as a team.

As family members define caregiving roles—through defining expectations—they give structure to the caregiving system. And some understanding of this structure (and its development) can help family members interact more effectively with professional care providers—as care needs increase and care duties mount.

The following tasks will help family members address here-and-now care issue—while laying the foundation for an adaptive, learning family system that meets shifting and mounting care challenges.

Task one: stepping in—the when question

The central question, in Phase Three, is not *whether* family members will step in. The question, instead, is *when* and *how* they will step in. The need to intervene—to begin assisting with specific tasks and activities of daily living—will inevitably occur. And difficult questions will inevitably arise. At what point is it most necessary and appropriate to step in? What is the process for stepping in? What are the potential consequences—for both the elder and the other family members?

We can't provide precise answers to these questions. But we believe that stepping in actions are usually driven by two concerns. First, family members feel an *obligation* to prevent their loved one from engaging in risky activities (driving, for example). Second, family members usually feel a *need* to compensate for a loved one's losses—to provide activities and forms of support that help the elder maintain a place in family life.

These stepping in actions cannot be avoided. And each action reaffirms a harsh reality: the elder has further declined and must further surrender some autonomy and freedom. Each action also drives home an insistent message, a decree that essentially says: *I am going to enter into your life in a new way—in a way that changes the rules of our relationship. I am going to make your business my business. And I am going to take charge of duties and responsibilities that were previously and exclusively yours.*

Stepping in actions are driven by various concerns. Family members might wish to safeguard the elder's safety. Or they might wish to maintain propriety—and prevent public embarrassment. Or they might simply wish to accomplish certain tasks more efficiently and conveniently—in order to conserve time, for example, or to maintain family routines.

These interventions are legitimate responses to "real-world" issues and concerns. With each step, the family "enacts" the caregiving role and assumes a new set of responsibilities. And, over time, the elder increasingly becomes a *care receiver*, and family members increasingly become *caregivers*.

In time, all the accumulated stepping in actions begin to constitute a caregiving system. *Thus, although the caregiving system may seem to emerge haphazardly and without conscious design, its development is, in fact, driven by specific stepping in actions that address short-term and long-term needs and concerns.*

Values and stepping in actions

The "when" question looms large in Phase Three, and the "timing" question is critical. At what point does the family take away car keys, for example, or take over shopping duties—or begin managing finances? These questions can prove perplexing, and family members may disagree about the timing and nature of the intervention.

For some family members, a stepping in action might represent a protective measure—a move that helps ensure the elder's safety (and perhaps the safety of other community members). For other family members, an intervention might represent a sign of disloyalty or even betrayal—an attack on the elder's autonomy and self-esteem.

Differing perspectives often reflect differing values—and differences in the ways family members prioritize their values. These differences and disagreements may require family members to reconsider and reprioritize their values. ("Do we mainly value our elder's freedom and autonomy?" "Or is safety our overriding value?") All decisions are value-laden. And, again, dialogue can help family members define and prioritize their values. It can help family members ensure that their decisions reflect their values—and that they're congruent with the family culture. And it can shape and guide intervention discussions and decisions.

Considering family members' interests

Family members possess both a right and an obligation to step in—to begin taking over tasks or portions of tasks. These actions are intended to help the impaired elder. But the interests of other family members—and all other stakeholders—must be taken into account.

Family members must closely consider the potential consequences of stepping in—and the hazards of *not* stepping in. And they must ask difficult questions. ("If we step in and something unexpected happens, how will we feel?" "If we don't step in and something unexpected happens, how will we feel?")

Moreover, family members must consider the duties that ensue from stepping in actions. If, for example, the family confiscates the car keys, who will assume driving tasks and other duties? Who will do the shopping and pay the bills?

When family members consider the needs, wants, interests, and values of all the stakeholders, they expand their perspectives. They avoid an overly-narrow focus on the elder. And they gain greater confidence in their decisions—even when decisions lead to unintended and unexpected consequences.

Considering the elder's interests

The question of whether to include the elder in family discussions comes up repeatedly in the early illness phases. We recognize the difficulties associated with bringing an elder into discussions that may lead to restrictions on his or her freedom and autonomy. Nonetheless, inclusion can provide some real benefits.

First, in the early disease stages, the afflicted family member usually possesses the ability to express competent opinions and to make useful observations. Through dialogue that includes the elder, family members may gain important insights into care approaches and quality of life issues.

Second, afflicted individuals throughout the course of the disease remain generally sensitive to the ways in which they are treated. They understand when they are being excluded—and when they are being ignored and devalued. To exclude an elder from critical discussions can temporarily relieve discomfort. But, for the elder, this exclusion can seem like an attempt to avoid honest and direct conversations—and to keep secrets.

Secrets can divide family members, damage relationships—and ultimately undermine a team approach to caregiving duties. A family that places a high value on openness and honesty will usually find ways to include the afflicted elder in most family discussions.

Using family dialogue to promote teamwork

Dialogue about stepping in actions can prove difficult and frustrating. And such dialogue may seem inefficient in the short-run. ("Why do we keep talking about this? Why don't we simply act?")

But dialogue allows all family members to offer their

unique perceptions, interpretations, and ideas—and to share their feelings. And when all voices—including the elder's—are included in the family conversation, family members gain greater access to the family "wisdom pool." They gain greater clarity and consensus. And, in our view, they ultimately make sounder and wiser decisions.

Each family will make the "when" decisions in its own unique way, and family members, in Phase Three, will find few clearly right and wrong answers. Decisions can lead to unwanted and unintended consequences, and the potential for finger-pointing, blaming, and second-guessing looms large.

Nonetheless when family members see Phase Three as a "trial and error" period—a transition period in which expectations, roles, and relationships are changing—we think they will lessen the potential for conflict and strain. When they listen carefully to all perspectives, and when they consider the interests of all family and community members, we think they will make wiser decisions. And we think they will feel more comfortable about the consequences of their decisions.

Task two: stepping in—the how question

The *when* question is followed quickly by the *how* question. That is, having decided to step in, family members next must develop some strategies for implementing their decisions—while maintaining the elder's dignity and self-esteem.

Again, difficult questions arise. How do we ask for the car keys? Should we ask—or should we simply confiscate them? How do we take over the checkbook? How do we deal with the loved one's resistance? How do we work with other family members?

In the face of difficult *how* questions, family members frequently think in terms of totally "taking over" certain tasks and entirely "taking away" certain rights and freedoms. And sometimes such action is required and justified. A car accident, for example, may require immediate confiscation of the car keys. Or serious financial mismanagement may require confiscation of the checkbook.

We think, however, that the "stepping in" actions can be viewed as a matching process—a process of matching the elder's specific capabilities to specific activities or specific tasks within an activity.

Matching capability to task

Alzheimer's victims lose their skills gradually—piece by piece over time. Losses initially show up in the ability to carry out complex activities. But, in the absence of other disabling conditions, Alzheimer's patients, in the early stages, usually retain the ability to carry out the smaller, simpler parts of an activity.

An afflicted elder, for example, may not retain the ability to plan and prepare an entire Thanksgiving dinner. But he or she may maintain the ability to complete smaller tasks—preparing the salad, for example, or basting the turkey. An elder may not retain the ability to fully manage personal finances. But he or she may be able to write out a check—or at least sign the check.

Thus, family members who are matching demand to capability must first see an activity as a set of *tasks*. Then, they can make a judgment (an estimation) about the tasks an elder can perform—and they can help the elder get started on a specific task.

This matching concept provides some large benefits— both for the elder and for the family. Through tailoring and modifying tasks and activities to match capabilities, family members help the elder maintain a sense of competence and a place in family life—and a sense of involvement in family routines and rituals.

Afflicted individuals, in the early stages, remain aware. They usually understand their impairments—although they may be reluctant to acknowledge them. And, indeed, they may find some relief in relinquishing tasks they can no longer perform well—so long as they can find other meaningful "replacement" tasks.

By matching tasks to capabilities, family members help safeguard the elder's dignity, self-esteem, and selfhood. They provide the elder with opportunities to succeed, and they relieve his or her sense of frustration and ineptitude. By matching tasks to capabilities, family members help the elder maintain a place in family life—and a sense of participation in family activities.

These matching actions also help family members. They often relieve feelings of disloyalty. And they help family members move away from "taking over" and "taking away" actions. Matching actions move family members toward a more positive approach, an approach that is not aimed solely at limiting the elder's activities—but that seeks to maintain the elder's involvement in family life.

Task three: foster the development of the caregiving system

Caregiving duties commonly fall upon one family member—frequently a spouse or a daughter. Family members don't usually "assign" these duties to a specific individual. Rather, one person generally assumes the early duties—and then, through a series of small steps, moves gradually into the primary caregiver role.

The primary caregiver may hold this caregiving role for months and years—sometimes until he or she reaches a point of physical and emotional exhaustion. In many cases, the primary caregiver, deenergized and demoralized, then hands off the duties to another family member—a kind of "tag team" maneuver that simply transfers care duties to another individual.

This approach may initially seem more efficient—it may seem to "make sense." But it can ultimately imperil the mental and physical well-being of the primary caregiver. And it can steer family members away from a cohesive and coordinated team approach that strives to share caregiving duties and to protect the well-being of all family members.

Thus, it's crucial, in Phase Three, for family members to discuss their expectations—to talk about *who* will do *what* and *when*. Without this kind of conversation (an expectations dialogue), some family members can feel "locked in" to a caregiving role—"trapped" in a role they can't negotiate. Others may feel "locked out" of a role—excluded from a meaningful place in the family caregiving structure. The consequence? Certain family members can find themselves deenergized and demoralized. And the family can find itself struggling to adapt—and to meet new challenges.

Thus, it's critical that family members, *in all phases,* maintain an ongoing dialogue about expectations and caregiving duties. Moreover, it's important for family members to see the caregiving system as a separate *system*—a system that interacts with the larger family system. This distinction helps family members see the importance of maintaining a vital family system, and it helps them see the ways in which a healthy family system supports the caregiving system.

Many factors influence the ways in which family members enter into caregiving duties. Some, for various reasons, can't participate in caregiving at all—but are able make other contributions to family life. Family conversations can help family members make conscious choices about their contributions. And, again, we think this dialogue can usefully revolve around boundary, structure, and culture issues.

Boundary

Boundary questions, as we've noted, relate to membership (who's in and who's out). And family members should strive, we think, to draw a clear boundary around both the caregiving system and the family system. Many factors can interfere with a family member's ability to participate in caregiving. Geographical separation, physical handicaps, other pressing family and work commitments, and lack of skills can interfere with the best intentions.

Thus, early conversations about boundaries are critical. These conversations help family members identify who's in and who's out of the caregiving system. And they help the family lay the foundation for future expansion of the caregiving system—as caregiving duties mount.

In the early stages of the illness, some family members may "sign up" for caregiving duties. Others may need to be "recruited." Our experience tells us, however, that most family members, in the early stages, will initially express a desire to contribute. General expressions of loyalty and support, however, do not always lead to concrete actions. Expressions of support ("We'll do whatever we can.") must be followed by specific commitments of time, energy, and resources. Moreover, these commitments should be made freely—and not driven by coercion or feelings of guilt.

Structure

With clearly established boundaries, with a clear sense of who's in and who's out, the family can then focus on the *structure* of the caregiving system—on expectations, roles, and relationships.

Early caregiving duties, in Phase Three, may be minimal, and, for some family members, conversations about expectations may lack urgency—or even necessity. But caregiving duties will inevitably increase over time. And family members will benefit greatly, we think, by focusing, in Phase Three, not only on here-and-now care concerns—but also on upcoming care duties and responsibilities. They will benefit from a dialogue that focuses on expectations: *who* will do *what* and *when* and *how.*

Well-defined expectations lead to well-defined caregiving roles. Clearly-defined caregiving roles give structure to the caregiving system—and lead to more effective and efficient forms of family care.

Conversations and dialogue about caregiving expectations and roles can prove difficult. But clear expectations can prevent and relieve strain. With clear expectations, family members know where they stand. And with clear roles, they can move forward—effectively anticipating problems and confidently addressing new challenges.

Culture

Many caregiving decisions reflect the family's long-standing and deeply-held values. And, as family members (through dialogue and discussion) make their decisions, they will find it useful to ponder those values—to reflect on them and to ask important questions.

Does our caregiving reflect the values of the family system? Does it reflect the family vision—and the ways in which we support one another? Does our caregiving consistently reflect our values? Or are we caught in value dilemmas? Should we rethink the importance we've attached to specific values? (Should we, for example, begin attaching more importance to safety needs—and less to autonomy and freedom needs?)

Family members, in Phase Three, face a complex challenge. They must find ways to integrate caregiving duties into family life—while maintaining other important activities (raising children, building careers). And they must maintain fundamental family values in the face of a disorganizing illness that holds the potential for undermining family routines and rituals—and for "taking over" family life.

When family members focus on the values that underlie family culture, we think they stay more connected to one another—and more connected to themselves (to who they are). When family members train conscious attention on the family's values, we think they better equip themselves to resolve perplexing care dilemmas. And they lay the foundation for an ongoing family planning process that anticipates both short-term and long-term care needs.

Task four: planning for change

Planning activities, in Phase Three, can seem like an unwanted and unnecessary burden. Planning conversations can prove difficult. They can exacerbate anxieties and tensions—and rekindle buried resentments and fears. And, in the absence of a major medical issue or other crisis, family members can find themselves steering away from long-term scenarios and painful (even unthinkable) "what if" questions. ("Why focus on potential problems when immediate problems seem so difficult?")

Nonetheless, early planning can ease decision-making in later stages of the journey, and it can provide some real short-term and long-term benefits.

First, early planning conversations allow the still-competent elder to express preferences about long-term medical treatments and difficult end-of-life issues. An elder, for example, might choose to appoint a proxy decision-maker, a family member who possesses legal authority to make medical decisions for the elder—when the elder is no longer able to make those decisions.

Moreover, early planning conversations help family

members formulate long-term financial plans in ways that protect the elder's assets—and safeguard family financial stability. For those with limited resources, planning discussions can help identify needed sources of assistance—financial and non-financial. And they can help identify the public and private criteria for obtaining help.

Early planning discussions help family caregivers match their caregiving abilities to specific care needs. And they help family members avoid a sense of being "locked into" caregiving roles—or "locked out of" desired roles (or any caregiving participation).

Most important, perhaps, early planning discussions help family members see themselves as a cohesive team that is pulling together and working toward common goals. Planning helps the family move from a *reactive* stance that responds only to the next problem or crisis into a *proactive* stance—into a stance that anticipates and responds to changing circumstances and emerging challenges.

Planning activities, in Phase Three, are an integral and critical component of the adaptive, learning family system. Increasing impairment in the elder will (sooner or later) force decisions upon the family. Family members who begin the planning process early will, in our view, develop a greater ability to identify options and to make deliberate and considered choices in all phases of the illness. And the family will find itself responding more effectively to immediate and upcoming care demands.

✦ CHAPTER EIGHT ✦

Phase Four:
The Chronic Care Phase

PHASE FOUR, THE CHRONIC CARE PHASE, IS MARKED by the impaired elder's increasing functional decline and dependence—and the need for constant (twenty-four-hour) vigilance. It's marked also by changing relationships—by changes in family members' relationship to the elder and to one another. And these changing relationships—together with mounting physical care duties—hold the potential for exhausting family life and threatening family well-being.

Family members keenly feel their elder's decline—and the ways in which their relationship to the elder is changing. They feel the grief and sadness that accompany loss and decline. And they mourn over the increasing loss of a familiar and treasured relationship.

Moreover, changes in the relationship with the elder reverberate throughout the family system—affecting all family relationships. And all these changes hold the strong potential for deenergizing family relationships and undermining family life.

The family's challenge, then, in Phase Four, is to maintain energy and vitality. And family members face the daily challenge of maintaining the emotional connections and the emotional energy that support family life—and that sustain family caregivers.

Let's look more closely at the relation between changing relationships and family vitality.

Issue one: maintaining family energy

Family caregivers, in Phase Four, face increasing strain. And family life—burdened by the elder's increasing losses and growing care demands—faces the threat of fatigue and ultimate exhaustion.

We've commonly associated this fatigue and exhaustion with the increasing and unrelenting *physical* care demands. But clinical and research evidence now tells us that the main source of exhaustion lies elsewhere. It derives mainly from the emotional loss and pain that accompany changing family relationships—changes in family members' relationship with their elder and with one another.

With increasing decline, the elder, in Phase Four, seems increasingly "there but not there"—physically present but increasingly psychologically and emotionally absent. The elder's personality and behavior, in Phase Four, is changing—often in disturbing ways. And family members see a loved one who (in some sense) seems familiar but who (in another sense) is beginning to seem like a stranger.

Pauline Boss calls this phenomenon *boundary ambiguity*. And, in her book *Ambiguous Loss*, she describes the various forms that boundary ambiguity takes—and notes its effects on Alzheimer's family caregivers.

The elder's steady decline and changing behaviors evoke feelings of grief and sadness—and other forms of emotional pain. And the emotional pain surrounding these changes can cause family members to step back—to begin distancing themselves from the elder and from one another. In an attempt to avoid painful daily reminders of their losses, family members can find themselves avoiding family interactions and activities.

The result? Emotional connections continue to loosen. Feelings of isolation develop. Family caregivers find themselves increasingly focused on caregiving duties. And family life begins to lose the energy and vitality that support and energize the caregiving system.

Thus the dilemma. When family members connect and interact, they experience emotional pain. When they seek to avoid pain—by disconnecting and distancing—they face emotional isolation and exhaustion.

This dilemma leaves family members with no seemingly good choices. They find themselves increasingly burdened (even captured) by exhaustion and emotional pain. And they find family life growing increasingly disorganized, demoralized, and deenergized—at a time when family caregivers need the support that only family life can provide.

Issue two: taking care of the caregiving system

Family caregivers, in Phase Four, also face a threat—the threat of increasing fatigue, isolation, and exhaustion. Caregivers find themselves devoting more and more time to care—and less and less time to themselves. And, in time, they can find themselves caught in a vicious circle. The more care they provide, the more exhausted they become—and the less time they find for renewal and replenishment. Without renewal and replenishment, and in the face of increasing care demands, they become less able to care for themselves—and less able to meet the increasing care demands.

These dementia care demands pose special challenges—and for some understandable reasons. First, this kind of caregiving is an open-ended experience. It's difficult to know when one is done—and difficult to know when one has done well. Thus, caregivers live in a constant state of uncertainty. And, without a clear sense of achievement, they find it difficult to maintain a sense of optimism and good feeling about their care activities.

Second, as the relationship with the elder continues to change, caregivers begin to lose a sense of give and take in the relationship. They lose "uplifts" and a sense of reciprocity—a sense that their efforts are understood and appreciated. With the elder's increasing inability to express appreciation (to say "thank you"), the relationship becomes increasingly one-sided. And many caregivers—giving and giving and ever giving—ultimately find that they have little left to give.

Third, caregivers can begin to feel isolated. Their lives can begin to revolve around caregiving, and caregiving can become their central and most involving daily experience. Friendships, interests, and usual activities drop away. Enjoyment and life pleasures fade and decline. And caregivers

can eventually find themselves bereft of any effective renewal and replenishment sources.

Caregivers need activities that renew and replenish them.
These activities safeguard their well being and ward off
exhaustion—a state of mind and body that carries serious
consequences. Exhaustion can undermine caregivers' sense
of security and competence—which can lead to feelings
of guilt and regret. Exhaustion can push enjoyment out of
caregivers' lives—which leads to even more exhaustion.

Thus the downward spiral. Caregivers lose activities
that renew and replenish them—and that energize them.
Without renewal and replenishment, fatigue builds—and
caregivers lose the interest and the ability to seek out renewal activities. Once begun, this spiral takes on a life of
its own—and becomes increasingly difficult to break.

This exhaustion can occur in any phase of the illness—
and at any level of care demand. Exhaustion, often insidious in nature, can interfere greatly with caregivers'
ability to care for themselves—to help themselves and to
accept help from others. Left alone, unheeded, exhaustion
inevitably builds—until, in many cases, it ultimately engulfs
family life.

The dangers in Phase Four loom large, and yet, we've
found that family members *can* find effective ways to navi-
gate through the difficulties.

In the tasks that follow, we will discuss some ways in
which the family can support the caregiving system through
maintaining its own energy and vitality. And we will discuss some ways in which the family can provide caregivers
with the renewal and replenishment resources they need to
carry them through this difficult phase.

Task one: understand and recognize the nature of strain

Family members, as we noted, often associate strain with physical care demands. They look for concrete ways to relieve these demands—and to reduce strain. But caregiving strain is a complex phenomenon. It derives from several sources—and it comes at families from several directions. And various forms can combine and interrelate in ways that exhaust family caregivers and deplete family life.

Intellectual

Caregiving is complicated work. Caregivers must constantly find ways to solve problems and formulate new care approaches. And, without the benefit of clear guidelines, they must constantly draw on their own knowledge, experience, and creativity.

Physical

Caregiving is hard work. The demands are constant and unrelenting. They require twenty-four hour vigilance. And caregivers face daily duties (bathing, dressing, toileting) that consume time and energy—and that allow little (if any) time off.

Emotional

Caregiving is sad work. Caregivers face daily signs of the elder's increasing decline and loss. And they must deal with a range of feelings—

sadness, worry, frustration, anxiety, depression, guilt. They must find ways to deal with these feelings—while managing the elder's emotional response to his or her impairments.

In the face of all these strains, one might think it logical to reduce each—and thus relieve the overall sense of strain. But these strains cannot be significantly reduced—by family members or by anyone else. Family members can't make the illness less confusing; they can't reduce the physical demands; and they can't make the experience less sad and worrisome.

Nonetheless, we know that some caregivers do better than others. Some caregivers stay more effective and optimistic—and more in charge of their lives. And we firmly believe the key lies in their ability to stay *energized*.

When family members understand that strain cannot be relieved through "fixing" problems and reducing care demands, they're more able to turn their attention elsewhere. They're more able to focus on the challenge of maintaining the caregiving system's energy through maintaining the system's organization—through supporting its boundary, structure, and culture.

Task two: support the caregiving system

The well-being of the caregiving system rests heavily on the well-being of the family system. And family caregivers rely greatly on the family system for support, renewal, and replenishment.

The family can more effectively support an organized

caregiving system. And an organized caregiving system can more effectively draw support from the family. In order to stay organized—and to "stay on top" of the illness—the caregiving system must attend to its boundary, structure, and culture. Let's once again look briefly at each.

Boundary

The collective efforts of individual caregivers constitute a caregiving *system*—a system that began in Phase Three with the early stepping in actions. In Phase Four, this caregiving system consists of all those individuals who contribute to care—both directly and indirectly.

Over time, with increasing care duties, this caregiving team can find itself struggling to meet the care challenges. And it can find itself asking whether it has sufficient resources—including sufficient people—to meet the caregiving demands.

As caregiving needs mount, the system must possess the ability to expand its boundary—and to bring others into the system. Family caregivers must be prepared to ask other family members for assistance—before strain and care demands engulf and exhaust them. And family members must be prepared to identify needs and step in with resources.

This "reaching out" and "reaching in" activity requires a conscious effort. Caregivers must be prepared to ask family members for help. And family members must stay sensitive to caregiving needs. They must stay informed and ready to assist—as demands increase.

But when caregivers "don't tell" and family members "don't ask," caregivers head toward fatigue and isolation.

And the caregiving system inevitably heads toward potential exhaustion.

Continual and ongoing communication helps family members overcome natural barriers and helps them address specific questions. "What are the caregiving needs?" Do we have a sufficient number of caregivers?" "Are we guarding against the threat of fatigue and exhaustion?" Families who maintain an adequate number of caregivers traverse Phase Four more effectively, and they more effectively avoid the threat of exhaustion.

Structure

As the caregiving system expands to include new people, it must continue to define, redefine, and organize individual caregiving roles. As family members step forward to provide help, they discover, through dialogue, caregiving needs and caregiver expectations. And they face some basic questions. "Who is willing and able to do what—and when?" How will we carry out the necessary tasks?" "What resources do we need?" "What kinds of help will help?"

Problem-solving activities, in Phase Four, revolve around the identification of needs—and the determination of tasks that will meet those needs. Some needs will relate directly to the care of the elder. Others may relate to the care of the caregivers—or other family members.

Family members must determine who will perform the caregiving tasks. And the family, in this phase, must again match task to capability. ("Who is able to do what?" Who is willing to do what?") As family members make their commitments, expectations become clarified, and the caregiving system becomes restructured.

This restructuring is an ongoing process. Alzheimer's disease, progressive and irreversible, constantly presents new care challenges. Caregivers may find that they've taken on overly burdensome tasks—tasks that they're unable or unwilling to carry out. Or they may find that they're able to shoulder additional tasks—more than they've estimated.

Roles, as we noted earlier, are defined by expectations ("Who will do what—and when and how?"). And the negotiation of expectations is an essential element in the redefining of roles and the restructuring the caregiving system. Expectations shape the ways in which family members relate to one another. And they help family members determine the ways in which caregiving duties and responsibilities will be conducted (who, what, when, how).

Family caregivers must constantly communicate their needs and their expectations—for themselves and for others. In the course of communicating needs, family members will find ways to support one another. They will find ways to stay connected and to relieve feelings of pain and loss. And they will operate as a cohesive team—staying abreast of changing needs and adapting to shifting demands.

Culture

All decisions are value-laden, and family care discussions inevitably reflect the family's values. The Phase Four complexities, however, can lead family members to differing views—and to disagreement about needed courses of actions. But even when family members disagree about proposed actions, they must keep in mind that they share certain core values. And their disagreements (a natural family phenomenon) may simply reflect a difference in the ways in which they've prioritized certain values (freedom vs. safety).

When making a decision, family members will find it useful to think about the values that underlie a specific goal—and to reflect on the ways in which a core family value can underlie differing strategies. This approach to decision-making can prove useful in Phase Four—a time when decisions grow inevitably more complex and clearly right and wrong answers grow increasingly elusive.

By staying focused on shared values, family members will maintain confidence in their decisions, and they will stay better connected and organized—even when decisions lead to unintended and unexpected consequences.

Shared values provide the "glue" that holds the family together. And a conscious focus on values, in Phase Four, can help family members stay organized and consistent—and supportive of one another. ("What are our goals?" "What do we most want to accomplish at this point?" "What do we most want to avoid?" "What parts of family life do we most want to preserve and protect?")

Staying organized

A focus on the caregiving system's *boundary, structure,* and *culture* can help family members keep the caregiving system organized—a critical element in Phase Four care activities. As we noted, family members are more willing and able to support an organized system—and to offer sources of renewal and replenishment. They are less able to support a disorganized system.

The caregiving system must also stay *energized*. It must draw energy from the family system. And to maintain this energy source, family members must strive to preserve family life. They must help caregivers maintain connections to family routines, celebrations, rituals, and problem solving activities. These activities help caregivers stay involved with family life and with one another—in a truly meaningful way. They help caregivers maintain morale and energy. And they help the family maintain cohesion and identity.

Task three: preserve family life

Family life supports the caregiving system and the emotional well-being of the caregivers. To cope more effectively—to protect against the threat of exhaustion—caregivers (and all other family members) must stay connected to a vital family life. But what do we mean by a vital family life? What's special about family life? What are its unique features?

Family life provides a structure and setting in which family members can grow and develop—and in which the caregiving system can stay grounded. Family life is special—and it is powerful. It provides forms of support and encouragement that family members simply can't find elsewhere.

We noted some of the unique features of family life in Chapter Two. Let's look briefly again at each feature and consider the ways in which each provides a unique form of support.

Stability

Families possess stable memberships. Other organizations come and go. But family connections endure. And the family endures—it maintains a powerful and enduring presence in the lives of all family members. Stability counts. It helps the family maintain cohesion, solidarity, and integrity. And a stable and vital family system provides a long-term foundation for caregiving efforts—and a safe harbor for all family members.

Intimacy

Lifelong ties allow for special forms of intimacy and connectedness. Family members possess special knowledge of one another— knowledge that no one else holds. Family members understand one another's needs, and they possess unique abilities to meet those needs. This special understanding is rooted in a shared history and set of shared values that are regularly affirmed in family rituals and celebrations.

Legitimacy

Family relationships hold a special status in society. Family bonds are considered sacred, and society grants special rights to the family group. Social institutions (the court system, for example) support family decisions and interfere with them only reluctantly. When family members reach agreement about a course of action, few will second-guess them—a powerful form of support in the face of tough choices.

Constancy

Families exist in time—they possess a past, a present, and a future. Family members are part of a long, enduring family journey—part of a group that endures across multiple generations. This group possesses a legacy from the past, and it possesses aspirations for the future. And family members look to this constancy for reassurance and support—for security and stability.

Age diversity

Families are among the most age-diverse organizations. Family life ranges across generations and life stages—up to five generations in some cases. Each generation possesses a unique and valuable voice. And these voices together—interacting with one another—generate a felt sense of energy. This energy strengthens both the caregivers and the impaired elder. And age diversity reminds family members that the family will go on—and that care must be seen within the context of the family's overall well-being and long-range goals.

These features, taken together, remind us of the unique nature of family life and the unique contributions of the family organization. To retain these unique features—and to maintain connections—family members must find ways to nurture and foster family life. They must pay specific attention to critical dimensions of family life—which include the family's day-to-day routines and rituals.

Through frequent communications (phone calls and visits), family members keep one another appraised of ongoing family events and activities. Through routines, rituals, and problem-solving activities, family members maintain connectedness. These interactions are most useful when they are frequent and diverse and meaningful—when they go beyond superficial interchanges. Enjoyable family activities remind family members of their common heritage and their unique relationships. And they help family members maintain a team approach to care issues.

Family events and activities all too often succumb to competing caregiving demands. But shared activities provide invaluable opportunities for family members to express pleasure in one another's lives—and to acknowledge one another's accomplishments. Shared activities help keep the family organized and energized. They help the family "stay bigger" than the illness—and "on top" of the illness.

The learning adaptive family system, in Phase Four, is more than a problem solving organization. It is a system that maintains emotional connections between and among family members. And it is a system that provides a sense of identity and set of shared values that support and sustain all family members.

The learning, adaptive family system, in Phase Four,

will find ways to maintain a vigorous and vital set of family activities. Through dialogue, it will find ways to meet various expectations. And through strong connections, it will maintain an environment that supports a strong, energized caregiving system. It will look to the future, anticipating the time when family members must begin to identify, seek, and obtain outside resources.

Task four: anticipate need for outside help

In the preceding tasks, we described some ways in which family members can stay connected to one another. And we described some approaches that can help the family stay organized—that can help family members keep the illness "in its place" and help caregivers avoid exhaustion and engulfment.

Family members, in Phase Four, face an additional task. They must anticipate further functional decline, and they must consider the point at which the family will require outside help.

Circumstances can change dramatically—and can suddenly and unexpectedly tax the family's resources and ability to manage. The adaptive, learning family system looks to the future, anticipating the time when it will need "outside" care services. It engages in contingency planning ("what if" conversations) that help the family prepare for events—expected and unexpected. And it "stays bigger" than the illness—prepared for the day when it must seek help.

Many family members reject the idea of outside help. Many place a high value on independence and autonomy—and feel more comfortable "going it alone." Others value privacy—and are reluctant to publicly acknowledge the presence of the illness. Still others find it difficult to admit "strangers" into the family's private and intimate world.

Resistance to outside help is understandable. Nonetheless, outside assistance is a legitimate part of family care. And an open attitude toward such care can provide some specific benefits.

First, it can make problems seem less catastrophic—and more subject to some kind of resolution. An understanding of the community's "safety net"—its set of formal and informal support services—can help family members feel less alone, less isolated.

Moreover, some focus on outside care resources can help family members understand the array of programs and services that are available—and it can lead them to some investigation of the resources. ("What are they?" "To what extent can they help?")

Early identification of resources can help family members obtain the right kind of help at the most appropriate and needed time. Moreover, openness toward professional assistance can relieve concerns about potential crises. And, in the face of unexpected problems (the primary caregiver's illness, the elder's suddenly worsening condition), knowledge of outside support can avert potential catastrophe.

For these reasons and others, it's important for family members, in Phase Four, to begin thinking about outside care assistance. Families who reject outside care— or who wait too long to obtain it—seem less able to maintain an organized, energized care system. Families who anticipate care needs—and who identify the ways in which "help can help"—seem more able to maintain stability in the face of change.

Most Alzheimer's families eventually need some kind of outside help. And a strong indication of family strength—of its ability to "stay bigger" than the disease—lies in its ability to reach out and find such help. In the next phase, Phase Five, we will examine the issues and tasks associated with identifying, contacting, and "bringing in" outside resources.

CHAPTER NINE

Phase Five:
The Shared Care Phase

PHASE FIVE: THE SHARED CARE PHASE, IS MARKED BY the recognition that mounting care demands are straining family resources and that the family must seek outside assistance. Family members, in Phase Five, have seen evidence that care demands are damaging family relationships and undermining family life. And they've reached the conclusion that "we can no longer go it alone—we need some kind of outside help."

Family resources vary, and each family will make its own determination about outside care in its own way—based on its own assessment of family wants and needs. The decision to seek outside help, however, signals the beginning of a major family system adaptation—the beginning or intensification of interactions with another system (the health care system) that will continue through the rest of the Alzheimer's journey.

The decision to seek help raises some basic questions. What kinds of help will help? What kinds are available? How do we bring outside help into the family caregiving system? How do we pay for it? What kind of help does the elder need? What kind do the caregivers need? Who can advise us?

Two broad concerns loom especially large: Why should we seek help? and When should we seek help? Let's look briefly at each.

Issue one: why seek help

In the face of increasingly burdensome care duties, some families still prefer to "go it alone," drawing only on family resources. Others choose to seek only the help of friends and other forms of informal support (self-help groups, for example). Many others, however, feel a need to reach out for professional help.

Unfortunately, many families see only one choice, only one form of outside help—placement in a nursing home. And many family members, repelled by the idea of nursing home care, delay their decision to seek *any* kind of assistance.

But outside help includes a broad array of services—a continuum of services and programs (formal and informal) that stretch between family care and nursing home care. And, with good planning and advice, many families are able to knit together an effective set of community programs and services—informal and formal.

Informal support

Informal support includes the assistance of friends, relatives, neighbors, community and religious organizations, self-help groups, and all the other individuals and groups who freely donate their services and support. In smaller communities, this informal support may be the only help available.

Formal support

Formal support includes programs and services designed specifically to meet dementia care issues and problems— and to address overall family concerns. Health care professionals, usually licensed by the state government, offer a structured set of services that meet specific needs. And they almost always assess a fee—although their payments (in part at least) may come from a government agency or from public grants.

The availability of formal and informal support services varies from place to place. Urban centers, for example, may offer a wider range of choices. But with a growing elderly population, and a growing need for Alzheimer's support services, choices are steadily increasing—even in smaller communities.

The decision to seek outside help represents a major *adaptation* in family life. And some family members may resist the idea. They may feel that outside help will undermine family control of family life. They may fear the undue influence of outside helpers. They may feel that they will be forced to surrender their own care approaches and to comply with the wishes of others. Some families simply fear the "privacy invasion," and they reject the prospect of "strangers" entering into the family's intimate and private daily routines.

Moreover, family members may hold differing perceptions about the elder's impairments—and may develop differing views about care needs. Disagreements can increase strain, and undue strain can lead to conflict. Conflict can further deplete family psychological and emotional resources. And unchecked disagreement and conflict can further exhaust and disorganize family life—and can ultimately damage family relationships. A thoroughly deenergized and demoralized family can reach a point at which *no* kind of "help can help."

Increasing care demands—developing slowly and insidiously over time—can eventually undermine caregiver health and erode family well-being. And families who delay the decision to seek outside help run the risk of inflicting permanent damage on family life. But when do family members know that it's time to seek help? How can they tell? How do they proceed?

Let's look more closely at the *when* question.

Issue two: when to seek help

The Phase Five question about when to seek outside help resembles, in some ways, the Phase Three question about when to intervene in an elder's life—when to "step in" and begin "taking over" tasks. In Phase Five, the question shifts from "When should we step into our *elder's* life?" to "When should we ask others (non-family members) to step into *our* lives and to begin sharing caregiving duties?"

Many family members find it difficult to define a precise point at which they should invite help into the family system. Individual family cultures and temperaments vary widely, and each family moves toward care decisions in its own unique way. Some families, as we've noted, are more open than others—and more ready to admit "outsiders." Others are more sensitive to privacy issues and more reluctant to invite "strangers" into family life. Indeed, some families see any kind of formal care as a last resort—the last option.

Many families look for "benchmarks"—for specific events and conditions that signal the need for help and that "legitimize" the decision to seek help. Family members, for example, might wait for a serious illness. Or they might wait for the elder to become incontinent—or seriously enfeebled.

These benchmarks *do* provide clear evidence that help is needed. But a focus on changes in the elder can steer attention away from other important considerations—from the need, for example, to consider caregiver and overall family well-being. As we've noted, caregivers can "burn out" over time. And family relationships can deteriorate as family members wait for the elder's illness to get "bad enough"— to reach the point at which family members can "justify" the need for outside help.

In the absence of a critical incident—an event that clearly signals the need for help—families tend to delay their search for help. Families who have been "carrying on" for months and years often feel that it's possible to carry on for one more day—and it usually is. But, again, delay can further stress family life. And prolonged stress can severely strain—even permanently damage—family relationships and family life.

Unfortunately, most families wait too long. They wait

for a serious problem or a crisis to develop (an elder's fractured hip, a caregiver's nervous breakdown). They wait for a serious "critical incident" that forces action. They wait until help is no longer a choice—but rather a need that is forced upon them.

Thus, it's critical, in Phase Five, for family members to look for signs of stress—to look for signals that help is needed. But what kinds of signs and what kinds of signals? We can't provide a formula, but we can offer some general guidelines.

In general, when communications among family members becomes strained and difficult, it is time for help. When emotional connections loosen, and family members find themselves less and less involved in each other's lives, it is time for help. When family members lose the ability to work as problem-solving team—and begin to go their own ways—it is time for help. When family routines and rituals begin to wither and fade, it is time for help. And when tension and discord begin to permeate family life, it is time for family members to seek help.

Family members who are considering (or seeking) outside help might wish to consider three basic questions: 1) How can outside help benefit the elder? 2) How can it benefit the caregivers? 3) How can it benefit the family?

The family, in Phase Five, must first determine how "help can help"—and then begin the process of seeking outside support. But the process of reaching out and establishing a partnership with outside professionals, programs, and services can prove complicated—and can bring difficulties into family life.

Let's look at some tasks that will help family members

identify and obtain outside help—and help them weave it into the family caregiving system.

Task one: acknowledge need for help

The first step in obtaining help is to acknowledge the need. And the decision to seek help must be (if possible) a *family* decision—a consensus decision that takes into account all perspectives. *Lack of agreement between and among family members can undermine an effective working relationship with outside helpers. And ongoing conflict and criticism can undermine and destroy the effectiveness of outside caregiving programs.*

Once more, dialogue can help family members achieve consensus. And the family dialogue, in Phase Five, can usefully focus, we think, on the benefits and burdens (or costs) of outside services. These costs go beyond financial "dollar" burdens. They can involve the loss of privacy and control—and the unwanted sharing of decision-making with "outsiders." The costs are real; they cannot be denied. But the benefits of outside care are many—both to the elder and to the family.

Benefits to elder

Experienced, professional Alzheimer's caregivers provide an array of services. Dementia care professionals can help family members understand and address specific Alzheimer's symptoms. Primary care professionals can monitor the elder's overall medical condition and can help keep function at an optimum level. Other medical professionals can evaluate and treat coexisting illnesses—and can generally help family members cope with various non-Alzheimer's health issues.

Occupational and physical therapists, social workers, and other specialists are equipped to assess and address the elder's living arrangements and lifestyle. These professionals can help family members structure the elder's daily activities and routines. And they can help the family develop strategies for safeguarding the well-being of both the elder and the caregivers. With effective preventive health care measures and quality of life enhancements, family members may extend the time that the elder can enjoy home care.

In addition, mental health professionals are equipped to evaluate the elder's psychological well being. They can identify emotional and psychological problems—depression and anxiety, for example. And they can provide counseling services that help both the elder and the other family members address emotional and behavioral issues.

Home health aides and adult day care providers provide special services. Day care services, for example, provide a structured environment and a set of specially adapted activities that offer respite to both the elder and the family caregivers.

Benefits to the family

Outside help benefits the family in several ways. Medical professionals can provide both educational and emotional support. They can help the family with the complicated work (problem-solving), the hard work (direct care), and the sad work (emotional demands). And they can provide assurance that the family is providing good care—that it is doing a good job.

Other professionals and services (home health aides and adult day care programs, for example) can provide respite. Support and self-help groups can provide new ideas, and they can provide information about the ways in which other families have coped (or are coping) with care challenges. These support groups can also help family members address feelings of isolation, loneliness, and failure.

Mental health professionals are equipped to address a range of emotional and psychological issues—including feelings of sadness, worry, and frustration. Family therapists, for example, can help the family develop more effective ways for communicating and achieving consensus around difficult issues. They can help family members achieve (or maintain) the kind of emotional closeness that safeguards family vitality and well-being.

In sum, outside help provides a range of benefits—for both the elder and the other family members. Outside assistance can support the elder's quality of life. It can help family members keep the Alzheimer's invader "in its place." And it can help the family stay vitalized and organized. Yet, many families find it difficult to acknowledge their need for help—and, perhaps, for some understandable reasons.

Barriers to acknowledging the need for help

A number of factors can interfere with the family's efforts to find outside assistance. The family, for example, may not fully understand its care needs. Or it may not understand all the services that are available—all the ways that "help can help." And, as we noted, even when family members conclude that help is needed, they often delay the decision to seek it. This kind of procrastination is understandable. But it's potentially damaging, and it's frequently related to some boundary, structure, and culture issues.

Family members, as we noted, may be reluctant to open up the family boundary and to bring "outsiders" into intimate family life. They may be reluctant to relinquish or redefine their caregiving roles—to change the caregiving structure. And they may be apprehensive about the ways in which outside help will affect the family culture and value system. ("Will outside help support our values?" "Will it take over our family life?")

Dialogue can bring barriers into the open—and can help family understand more clearly how "help can help." Family conversations can help family members work through barriers and reach a consensus that all stakeholders (the elder, the caregivers, and the family) can benefit from outside assistance. With this acknowledgement, family members can then move more effectively to the other Phase Five tasks.

Task two: identify and explore available health services

Having acknowledged the need for help, family members next must begin to define the kind of help they need—and to identify the kind that's available. Community resources vary, and the range of Alzheimer's services can vary widely from community to community. Basic questions arise. What kinds of help will help? Where should we begin?

Who can help us identify Alzheimer's care resources? Who can guide us through the health care maze?

The identification of care needs begins in the home. And it begins, we think, with an inventory—with a list that defines family members' care goals. With this list in hand, family members can then begin defining their wants and needs.

A few simple questions can begin the process of identifying specific care needs. What, for example, are the "sticking points" in the day? In the daily care routine, what are the most troublesome points? What are the care tasks that seem most burdensome and fatiguing—and just plain irritating? What parts of everyday family life have been "taken over" by the illness. Which parts do family members miss the most? Which issues seem most difficult to discuss? Which seem most challenging—even overwhelming?

Family caregivers can usually answer these questions with some precision. And, with some reflection, they can then begin to prioritize their needs—and to identify the ways in which "help can help" at specific points in the day. With this knowledge, caregivers can then begin the process of matching care needs to available community health care resources.

Task three: initiate contact with health care system

It's helpful, we think, to view community care resources in terms of a *system* of care and a *continuum* of care. Health programs and services stretch across a continuum—each addressing special needs, And, in time of need, family members may find themselves moving across the continuum of care—moving from place to place in the system as care needs change and evolve.

The continuum of care contains an array of services and programs—including home care programs, day care programs, hospitals, multi-specialty clinics, rehabilitation centers, and nursing homes. And the family, in Phase Five, faces the task of identifying the available services within the continuum—and then choosing the appropriate "entry point."

These entry points may not always be obvious, and the complex health care system can sometimes prove bewildering. But help is available. Case management professionals and other professionals—social workers, case managers, and nurse clinicians, for example—can help family members identify appropriate services and help them find an appropriate entry point.

Family members may find their initial entry point unsatisfactory—or at least uncomfortable. And they should feel free to find another entry point along the continuum of care—another service or health professional to whom they can effectively relate and with whom they can develop a meaningful and satisfying relationship.

For many families, the best entry point into the care system is through a primary medical care professional. The family may have had a long association with a primary care physician or nurse—an association that gives the professionals a broad understanding of the family's experience and a special understanding its unique wants and needs. These primary care professionals provide a stable anchor. They can offer sound advice about care options, and they can help family members work through the "health care maze."

Task four: establish relationship with health care system

After making an inventory of family needs and exploring the available services, it would seem that family members need only match services with needs—a seemingly simple task.

Our experience tells us, however, that the process of obtaining help is a bit complicated. And it's critical, we think, for family members, in Phase Five, to understand that they are not simply purchasing services. *They are establishing (or should be establishing) a relationship with the health care providers and their organizations—a relationship that may continue over months and years (even, in some cases, decades).*

Thus, family members and their helpers benefit from a "good match"—from a compatible and comfortable relationship. The process of establishing a good relationship, resembles in some ways a "courtship"—a "getting to know you" process that allows both parties to develop solid mutual understandings. A good "courtship" leads often to a good "marriage"—a match rooted in shared values and common visions about care goals and approaches. A poor "courtship" can lead to a disconnected and tense relationship—and to ongoing conflict and turmoil.

As we noted, some families find it difficult to ask for help. And too many families wait too long. They wait for a crisis, and they find themselves making decisions and establishing relationships in a crisis state—in emergency circumstances that don't allow for a proper "courtship" and a sufficient getting acquainted period.

Early planning and early identification of suitable services can ease the transition into shared care. Smooth interactions between family caregivers and outside helpers can pave the way for a partnership—for the joining of unique skills and knowledge that help both professionals and family members reach their goals.

Clear goals help professionals and family members move toward a cooperative and collaborative relationship. Conversations about goals help both family members and helpers clarify their expectations—for themselves and for one another. And they help both sides identify shared values. Through clarifying expectations, defining goals, and prioritizing values, family members will more effectively maximize the benefits of shared care—while minimizing its burdens.

Alzheimer's care poses severe challenges—both to family members and to outside helpers. But firm and supportive relationships between family members and their helpers provide an invaluable base of support. And shared-care partnerships—resting on a firm foundation of trust and understanding—can help family members optimize their resources and safeguard family life.

For many families, however, care demands eventually begin to outstrip both family *and* outside care resources. Many families eventually find it difficult, if not impossible, to continue an effective home care program. And many must eventually turn to a long-term care option—the subject of our next discussion.

CHAPTER TEN

Phase Six:
The Nursing Home Phase

PHASE SIX, THE NURSING HOME PHASE, IS MARKED BY the recognition that home care is reaching its limits—and that nursing home care is now a viable option. Not all families will choose nursing home care. But most families, at some point, will consider nursing home care—or some other kind of long-term care. And many families will ultimately decide that their elder *ought* to be placed in a long-term care facility.

But what do we mean by *ought*? At what point does the family decide that placement *ought* to occur—that it is the best option?

It's difficult to define the precise moment at which a family should begin thinking about nursing home care. Some families reach the decision when an "expert" (usually a physician or, perhaps, an informed family member) tells them that the "time is now." Other families make the decision when they can no longer "carry on"—when the elder's behavior and health problems simply exceed family caregiving capabilities.

Each family will make its placement decision in its own unique way—based on its own unique circumstances and needs. We think, however, that the family can profit from a "benefits and burdens" calculation—from a careful weighing of the benefits and burdens associated with each form of care (home care vs. facility-based care).

This kind of calculation, in our view, can foster consensus and ease decision-making. But it must take into account the needs and wishes of all the stakeholders—the *elder,* the *family caregivers,* and the overall *family system.*

For some, it may seem a bit strange to speak about the benefits of nursing home care. For many family members, nursing home care seems like the worst alternative—the least attractive option. But institutional care can provide large benefits—for both the elder and the other family members. And a productive "benefits" discussion can help family members move toward a decision in a careful way—and in a calm, non-crisis atmosphere.

Let's look more closely at issues surrounding the *why* and *when* questions.

Issue one: why seek nursing home care

As we noted, many families find it difficult even to contemplate the nursing home placement decision. For many, nursing home care seems like the last possible option—a "bad," unavoidable, unwanted choice that is ultimately forced upon them. Many family members fear the subject. They consider placement discussions a "taboo" subject—a sign of disloyalty. Even when family members secretly lean toward nursing home care, they often find it difficult to introduce the subject into the family dialogue.

The reluctance to consider nursing home care is understandable. For some family members, placement can seem like a form of abandonment—a disloyal and heartless act. Many nursing homes have poor reputations. And many family members feel that others will blame them—even castigate them—for "putting their loved one away."

But without early and open discussion, family members can find it difficult to reach an informed decision. And they can ultimately find themselves facing placement decisions that are forced upon them (by serious illness, for example)—and for which they are ill-prepared.

Thus, many families approach nursing home care with little preparation—and with little understanding of its benefits. And many families continue to consider nursing home care the last option—the last possible choice.

The nursing home decision *is* laden with emotion, and contemplation of placement can add to already strong feelings of grief and sadness. Nonetheless, it's useful for family members to recognize some essential "truths" about nursing home care—and about the issues surrounding the decision to seek such care.

The decision to consider or seek nursing home care does not mean that the family can no longer provide care. The decision simply means that the benefits associated with nursing home care significantly outweigh the burdens. And this burden-benefit equation can provide a foundation for family dialogue and discussion—a way of introducing the subject into the family dialogue.

Family members can usefully raise some central questions: What are the physical, psychological, and emotional *burdens* of continued home care—to the elder, to other family members, and to family life? And what are the *benefits* and *burdens* of nursing home care? How can nursing home care enhance the well-being of all family members—and safeguard the well-being of family life?

These kinds of questions move family members into a more productive stance. They move family members away from a consideration of family *limits* and a sense of failure—and toward a more useful discussion of *benefits*. They help family members see placement as a *choice*—a freely-made decision that rests on a consideration of *benefits*.

Let's look at a few of these nursing home care benefits.

Benefits to the elder

Nursing homes possess dementia care expertise. Forty to sixty percent of *all* nursing home residents labor under some form (or degree) of dementia—usually Alzheimer's disease. And nursing home staff members understand the dementia care challenges. Professional nursing staff members are trained to identify and address specific dementia symptoms and behavior problems. And many nursing homes provide ongoing training programs for staff members who work with dementia patients.

Moreover, many nursing homes provide special care units for Alzheimer's patients. These units offer an ongoing set of programs and activities that provide stimulation and companionship. These special programs and activities—together with the contributions of an experienced staff—help create a caring and comfortable environment. With structured routines, the elder's "here and now" reality becomes more predictable and manageable.

In addition, the experienced nursing staff is trained and equipped to monitor, assess, and manage an array of co-existing medical conditions (heart problems, diabetes, infections, for example). Nursing professionals are able to evaluate and assess dementia patients who cannot effectively communicate their symptoms and needs. These professionals can monitor for symptoms of illness and identify health problems early on—when they can be more easily treated.

Benefits to the caregivers

Family caregivers can, over time, find themselves "organizing" their lives around the illness—devoting themselves to the elder's care needs while neglecting their own needs, wants, and interests. Caregivers can find themselves "giving and giving" to the point of exhaustion—and even illness.

Nursing home care relieves family caregivers of the daily physical care demands. Relieved of these daily (sometimes "engulfing") demands, family caregivers are more free to focus on the elder's psychological and emotional needs. They are more free to offer the unique forms of assistance—the nurturance and support—that only they can provide.

Benefits to the family

Nursing home care allows family members to step back from the illness and to begin reclaiming parts of family life that have been "taken over" by the Alzheimer's "invader." It provides assurance that care needs and medical evaluations are being handled by trained professionals. And it allows family members to begin reinvesting in neglected parts of family life.

Moreover, nursing home care can often relieve the family's sense of isolation. It provides opportunities for family members to associate with others who are dealing with similar issues and who are traversing similar ground—the Alzheimer's terrain.

Nursing home care *does* carry certain burdens. The elder may resist the move to unfamiliar surroundings. Caregivers may feel that they've relinquished control of their elder's care. And, for many families, nursing home care may not, in fact, be the best option.

But when family members carefully consider both the benefits and burdens of nursing home care, we think they make better choices. We think they make decisions that are more congruent with the values and goals of the entire family. And, if nursing home care is their choice, they move more easily to the "when" question.

Issue two: when to seek nursing home care

As we noted, many families recoil from the idea of nursing home placement. And, in our experience, most families wait too long. They wait too long to initiate the family dialogue and discussion. And they wait too long to make the placement decision.

Family members tend to ask the question, "Can we continue to provide care and to keep our loved one at home?" And the answer to the question is often, "Yes, we can continue—for another day, another week, another month. Perhaps we can continue indefinitely."

Moreover, family members may wait for a "critical incident"—an accident or a severe medical problem, for example, that seems to take the decision "out of their hands." But family members who wait for a critical incident may find themselves making placement decisions in a climate of crisis—in stressful circumstances that leave little room for careful and deliberate planning.

Barriers to seeking care

The decision to consider nursing home care is laden with emotion, and the barriers to seeking such care—or even discussing it—can prove formidable.

Nursing home care still carries a certain social stigma, and many families still see nursing home placement as one step away from "prison placement." Many families feel that nursing home placement represents a form of "surrender"—the abandonment of family obligations and the betrayal of a beloved elder. Even when family members truly accept that nursing home care is the best choice, the decision still carries feelings of guilt and remorse.

Moreover, many family members cannot bring themselves to see nursing home care as another step in the care process—another step along the continuum of care. Many tend to see nursing home care as simply one more "step toward death"—the last stop in a dreadful journey. And the grief surrounding placement can prove overwhelming.

Grief and sadness often surround the nursing home decision, and family members understandably find reasons to avoid the placement issue. They find it difficult to initiate a nursing home dialogue—and to begin discussing placement. But the family discussions are critical. They help ensure good decisions and a smooth placement, and they foster a team approach to nursing home care.

Through dialogue, family members can overcome barriers to discussing placement—and can establish a process for making a planned transition into nursing home care. In the tasks that follow, we will lay out the process for making that transition—and for initiating and maintaining a relationship with the nursing home facility.

Task one: anticipate and plan

Nursing home placement represents a major event in family life—a major step in the Alzheimer's journey. But, as we noted, most families wait too long to initiate a dialogue and discussion about nursing home care—and they wait too long to make the transition into nursing home care.

Moreover, family members who have not developed some kind of contingency plan often find themselves making the decision in a crisis atmosphere—under pressures that early planning might have prevented.

Alzheimer's families possess opportunities to carefully consider the benefits of nursing home care—even early in the illness. The chronic nature of Alzheimer's disease—its slow and steady progression—gives family members time to inform themselves about long-term care, to explore long-term care options, and (if the decision is made) to develop a transition plan.

Moreover, early dialogue and planning allow the elder to participate in the decision-making process. Elders in the early disease stages still possess decision-making abilities. They're concerned about the ways in which their care will affect family members and family life. And many possess firm opinions about the kind of care they wish to receive—and where they wish to receive it.

Early family conversations can begin, we think, with some "what if" questions. ("What if the elder's physical condition suddenly deteriorates?" "What if caregivers can no longer continue?") Contingency plans and emergency planning can ease worries—and can promote the dialogue and flexibility that leads to effective decision-making.

Early dialogue helps family members bring the nursing home option into the open. It helps the family understand the benefits and limitations of continued home care—and the potential benefits of nursing home care. And it may help the family move more easily toward consensus—and toward specific "when" and "where" conversations.

Nursing home care and family values

The nursing home decision is tied closely to the family's values and goals. And family dialogue, we think, should begin with some examination of care goals—and the values that underlie those goals.

Values guide choice and action. The ways in which

family members assess the benefits and burdens of nursing home care and home care rest greatly on the ways in which they define and prioritize their values. And a firm understanding of the family's values (together with clear statements about desired courses of action) help ensure that placement decisions are congruent with family values.

Family dialogue facilitates effective family decision-making, and it can lead to various decisions. Through dialogue, family members might conclude that continued home care is still the best option—and that they should stay the course. Or they might conclude that nursing home care—at some point—is a viable option. Or, as dialogue and discussion continues, family members might decide that placement needs to occur soon—or perhaps immediately.

When family members conclude that nursing home care *may* be required, they must then begin the process of finding a suitable facility and preparing for the transition. This process involves a series of specific steps.

Gather information.

The first step is to identify the available facilities—and to determine the nature of the care they provide. Family members should also inquire about the nature of the waiting list (if one exists).

Nursing home information can be obtained from various sources. Community, religious, and health care organizations provide information about long-term care and other forms of elder care. Social workers, primary care physicians, public agencies, and local Alzheimer's associations can also provide information about nursing home availability—and about the reputations, services, programs, and capabilities of specific facilities.

Informal sources of information can prove helpful. Friends, relatives, and associates—many of whom may have had direct experience with nursing home care—can often provide valuable advice and counsel. They can help shape initial decisions and help lay the groundwork for other decisions. For some families, location and proximity might be the critical factors. For others, reputation and cost might be the primary factors.

Visit and evaluate nursing homes

With a list of facilities in hand, family members can begin exploring specific possibilities. Family members can gain a strong impression of the nursing home culture and environment through simple visits. They might, for example, observe the physical structure of the facility. Is it well-maintained? Does it have a pleasant appearance? Is it clean—and free of odors?

Family members can also observe the interactions 1) between and among staff members and the residents, 2) between and among staff members, and 3) between and among residents. Do staff members seem engaged and happy? Are residents interacting with staff members—and with each other? Are supervisory staff members present on the units? Are all individuals (staff members and residents) being treated courteously and respectfully?

Through observing these interactions, family members can gain an overall sense of the organizational culture and the ways in which the nursing home allows and encourages free and open interrelationships. And they gain a sense of how the family system interacts with the nursing home system. Does the nursing home culture match the family culture? Do family members feel comfortable with nursing home staff members?

Reaching consensus

Consensus is critical. And families can gain greater consensus through allowing and encouraging *all* family members to participate in information gathering and facility visits. Consensus strengthens a team approach and helps avoid recriminations, conflicts, and second-guesses—all of which only add to existing pain and guilt.

After gathering information and considering the benefits of nursing home care, the family (through dialogue and discussion) must then weigh their options, prioritize their choices, and reach a consensus decision. ("Should we place now?" "Or should we wait—and continue the home care program?")

If family members, after having carefully considered the "why," "when," and "where" issues, make the decision to place their elder in a facility, they must them address the "how" issue—and prepare for the move.

Task two: make the move

The transition into nursing home care is usually a process that occurs over time, and family members usually have time to prepare for the placement event. Nonetheless, "moving day" is a hard day and a traumatic day—a difficult and exhausting day. Placement is a major event in both the Alzheimer's journey and the family journey. And it represents the beginning of a major family system *adaptation*.

Family members benefit, we think, from making the move a "joint venture"—an experience that includes as many family members as possible. This kind of family gathering (not unlike the gatherings that occur at marriages, births, graduations, and deaths) makes the event a kind of family ritual—a significant piece of family history that all family members can later reflect upon.

Moving day can also be a traumatic experience for the elder. Large and noisy crowds can overstimulate an afflicted elder. But the presence of family members can relieve and elder's upset and turmoil. And the presence of family members during the early weeks of nursing home care sends a powerful statement of support to both the elder and the nursing home caregivers.

Nursing home staff members can usually assist with the transition. Their experience with previous admissions gives them insight into the difficulties and challenges surrounding "moving day." Family members should feel free to ask these professionals for suggestions and guidance.

Admission process

The admission process begins with some pre-admission "paperwork" and other "bureaucratic" activity. Nursing home admission personnel can usually assist with the paperwork tasks—and can provide information about the admission procedure. They can describe care policies and procedures. And they can help the family identify the individual (family member or otherwise) who will be responsible for making financial and medical decisions.

At the point of admission, information about the elder is processed and delivered to the appropriate nursing station. Staff members help the elder get settled in his or her room. They mark belongings, order medications and supplies, and begin orientation to the unit. The multidisciplinary staff then takes over—completing assessments, meeting with the family members, and carrying out other required admissions tasks.

Family members may be able to prepare the elder for the move—but they may not. There may be little to explain and little point in trying to reason with the afflicted loved one—who may not comprehend the event. Nursing home staff members possess wide knowledge about placement issues. And they can guide the family through the "moving day" process—including the difficult "goodbye" process.

The paperwork and the moving procedures constitute the "moving day" tasks. But family members, on moving day, face some emotional challenges. And many experience a complex (sometimes conflicting) set of emotions: sadness at leaving the elder in the care of others together with a sense of relief—a sense that daily caregiving duties have finally ended. Mutual support among family members is critical at this point, and family cohesion and dialogue can greatly ease the tensions and difficulties surrounding "moving day."

Task three: establish partnership with nursing home staff

Family members can (and should) expect to establish a relationship with the nursing home system—and with the individual nursing home staff members. This partnership rests on the premise that all parties have a useful and legitimate role to play. And it develops through dialogue that addresses both the expectations of the family *and* the expectations of the nursing home staff.

A collaborative relationship—a partnership based on trust and understanding—can enhance the decision-making process. It can help the family and the staff face difficult care issues. And it can help ensure satisfactory approaches to complex and perplexing problems.

Unlike the home care system, with its more informal and intimate relationships, the nursing home organization is a complex system—organized mainly around formal roles and professional relationships. And its routines tend to be less flexible than family routines—more set and stable.

For many family members, nursing home care can initially seem formal and "strange." Nursing home staff members can seem like "experts"—and family members can feel like "customers." The family—despite its caregiving experience and knowledge of the elder—may initially feel "locked out" of a caregiving role. And family members may feel that they've come to the end of the journey—even though they still have much to contribute.

Moreover, family members may see nursing home placement as a "tag team" event—a "hand-off" that leaves little opportunity for continued family involvement. But this way of looking at placement can undermine the family's opportunity to establish a *partnership* with the nursing home system. And it can close off opportunities for extending family care into the nursing home setting.

The nursing home staff brings professional expertise to dementia care. But the family possesses intimate knowledge of the elder—a keen understanding of the elder's temperament and personality, likes and dislikes, peculiarities and eccentricities. Both forms of knowledge—family knowledge and nursing home care expertise—are critical. And, through dialogue, both can be joined in ways that foster a partnership between the family system and the nursing home system.

Relieved of physical care burdens, family members are more free to deliver the unique forms of care and support that only they can provide. That form of care is greatly enhanced when both systems—the family system and the nursing home system—recognize the unique and invaluable knowledge that family members bring to care goals and activities.

Systems and relationships

To begin an effective partnership, it's useful to think first in terms of two systems (the family system and the nursing home system) coming together in mutually beneficial and agreed upon ways. And, once again, it's useful to reflect on the familiar elements of a system—its boundary, structure, and culture.

Family members must first clearly state their intent to remain involved in the elder's care. And they must work closely with the nursing home staff in ways that allow the facility to open its *boundary* and to accept family assistance.

Moreover, family members must establish a dialogue that allows the expression of expectations and that helps define roles and relationships—the *structure* of the newly organized system of care.

A successful system partnership rests also on the ability of the two systems (family system and nursing home system) to effectively communicate their expectations and to work toward mutual goals—goals that are based on congruent *values* and an understanding of the family *culture*. Open discussion of these values and care goals can foster a sense of partnership and can ultimately enhance care.

Interactions between family members and staff members

Interactions between the family and the facility can occur informally through conversations with staff members. And they can occur in more formal settings—at family/staff conferences, for example.

Informal interactions with staff members help family members establish and cement relationships—and they benefit both staff members and family members. Through effective interactions, staff members gain valuable support and feedback from family members. And family members gain the opportunity to share their caregiving experience with the staff and to provide an overall picture of the elder—an overall sense of who the elder is and what he or she has accomplished.

Formal care conferences are mandated by regulations—

and may include both supervisory and nursing staff members. Family members should expect to participate in these conferences and to freely share their perspectives on care goals and strategies.

Collaborative relationships support nursing home staff members. A supportive family system enhances nursing home care and may reduce the potential for conflict and adversarial relationships. And collaboration can begin with a simple step—*the sharing of the elder's life history.*

Family members possess unique forms of knowledge about this history—and about the elder's personality and values. When they share this knowledge, they communicate the elder's "specialness" and selfhood. They paint a picture that helps staff members understand and appreciate the elder's life experience.

A collaborative partnership can also help family members—and nursing home staff members—establish care goals that are consistent with the policies and culture of the nursing home, that recognize the autonomy of the patient and the values of the family, and that recognize the importance of the medical professionals' integrity.

To facilitate the partnership, the nursing home must know the individual who is legally authorized to make health care decisions for the incompetent elder. (The nursing home may request a copy of the living will or durable power of attorney.)

To further facilitate communication, the family might wish to designate an individual with whom the nursing home can effectively and quickly communicate. This individual (an information "conduit") can then communicate information to other family members.

The family might also wish to identify a nursing home staff member (a "point person") with whom family members can communicate. Effective communication enhances the partnership—and the system of care—that the family and the nursing home have created.

Task four: accept and recover

With placement, family members (within a period of hours and days) can find themselves moving from a life centered on daily care to a life devoid of such duties. And this period can, for many family members, seem like a "void"—a confusing blend of "finishing" and "beginning." Family members can feel that something, somehow, is "missing" from their lives.

Nursing home placement represents a major family system adaptation. And it requires, like other adaptations, a restructuring of family life. Nursing home placement relieves family members of the daily home care demands. But family members may, during this transition period find themselves struggling to establish new caregiving roles—and new ways of structuring their daily lives. Following placement, many of the old "rules" and expectations no longer apply. And family members find themselves facing a "new world"—and a new set of rules and expectations.

During this transition period, family members can find themselves grieving the "loss" of the elder—as they strive to develop ways for moving into nursing home care activities. But this period also provides opportunities for family members to reflect on their achievements—to take stock of the ways in which they have provided a caring and loving environment for their elder. This kind of reflection can help family members find meaning and new directions.

Family members can benefit from establishing a dialogue that addresses the family's future. Where are we going? How will we now meet our goals—unencumbered by the daily demands of Alzheimer's care? How will we handle this new-found freedom?

Family members might wish to focus on two themes: What is the nature of the journey we have been traversing? and What will be the nature of the journey on which we are now launched? These kinds of conversations can help the family manage the nursing home transition. And they can help family members prepare for the end-of-life phase—the end of the Alzheimer's journey.

CHAPTER ELEVEN

Phase Seven:
The End of Journey Phase

PHASE SEVEN, THE END OF JOURNEY PHASE, IS MARKED by the family's sense that the elder is dying—and that death seems imminent. Previously effective medical treatments seem now to bring only temporary improvements. And family members, in Phase Seven, face an inescapable reality: the afflicted elder is not "coming back"—life is ending. And the family Alzheimer's journey is nearing an end.

This end-of-life phase evokes a mix of feelings—sadness and grief, for example, coupled with a sense of relief. And it presents two major challenges: 1) how to ensure a "good death" for the elder and 2) how to ensure closure for caregivers and other family members. But what exactly constitutes a good death? And what constitutes closure for an Alzheimer's family?

Issue one: dying well

We tend to think of death as an entirely unwelcome event. And, for many family members the notion of a "good death" may seem a bit strange. Nonetheless, in recent years the "dying well" movement has gained increasing acceptance and millions of Americans have expressed interest in a good death—an end-of-life experience that focuses on comfort and dignity and adherence to previously-stated wishes.

Society respects the right of competent adults to make decisions for themselves—and to accept or reject treatments. But when elders are unable to make decisions (because of dementia, for example), the legal and health care systems turn often to the family—the group most capable of making difficult end-of-life decisions.

Alzheimer's family members are often surprised to learn that they are expected to participate in end-of-life decisions—and to address questions that go beyond medical expertise and judgement. Again, as in previous phases, difficult questions arise. Should we, for example, prolong life—at all costs? Or should we strive mainly to ensure the loved one's comfort, dignity, and quality of life? What constitutes a "good death" for the elder? What decisions would the elder make—if he or she could decide?

The elder's previously stated wishes (a living will, for example) can assist. But early discussions and documents—helpful as they are—can't possibly anticipate all end-of-life events and circumstances. And society turns often to the family for end-of-life judgements.

Families who decline the decision-making role will find decisions being made solely by health care professionals. These professionals carry out their professional obligations. But they are often constrained by legal and ethical standards that emphasize the prolongation of life—but that may result in needless suffering.

A "good death" for the impaired elder, then, means a death the elder would choose—if he or she were able to decide. And, for the family, it involves end-of-life decisions that are congruent with the elder's wishes and values.

Family members are uniquely positioned to interpret and represent these wishes and values. And they are uniquely equipped to help the elder experience a "good death," one that helps ensure comfort and dignity—and that helps bring closure to the Alzheimer's journey.

Issue two: finding closure

For non-Alzheimer's families, an elder's death normally evokes feelings of sadness and grief—and a sense of loss. These feelings linger for a while. But, in time, family members usually find closure and take up their lives again— moving forward and pursuing their interests and goals.

For Alzheimer's families, closure is a more difficult and complex issue. Closure for the Alzheimer's family involves not only a "goodbye" to the elder—but also a "letting go" of the illness. It involves a recapturing of the elder that family members once knew—before the illness. And it involves a reclaiming of family life.

For Alzheimer's family members, grieving begins early and continues throughout the Alzheimer's journey. Pain and sadness accompany all phases of the Alzheimer's journey. And even though the end can feel like a welcome change, it can also leave a void—an empty space in family life that must be filled. Family members feel this void. And to fill it, they must make a conscious effort to reclaim family life—to reorganize and reinvest in family life and family relationships.

In the tasks that follow, we will describe some ways in which family members can help ensure a good death for the elder and achieve effective closure for themselves.

Task one: make end-of-life decisions

For many American families, death remains a taboo subject. We fear it; we deny it; we even joke about. And then, when it approaches, we feel unprepared. We turn away—isolating loved ones and rejecting opportunities to fully explore this deep and complex human experience.

For Alzheimer's families, the end-of-life experience poses special challenges. They must make decisions for a demented elder who can no longer communicate his or her wishes. *And they must begin to change the nature of their medical goals.*

In Phase Seven, *curing*—the attempt to restore function and health—is no longer the major medical goal. *Caring*—the attempt to ensure comfort, dignity, and quality of life—is now the chief goal. And family members, in Phase Seven (the end-of-life phase) must begin to make sound *caring* decisions—decisions that focus primarily not on *curing* but on comfort and dignity.

These "caring" decisions can prove difficult. But family members, with their deep understanding of the elder's values, are uniquely equipped to guide this kind of medical decision-making. They have observed the elder's decisions over a lifetime. And they are uniquely positioned to make health care decisions that reflect the elder's values—and that are consistent with the elder previous decisions (over the course of a lifetime).

As we noted, certain legal instruments *can* help family members carry out the elder's wishes. A *living will,* for example, can communicate some broad wishes and can provide *some* guidance. But these living wills, helpful as they are, remain imperfect instruments—they can't possibly address all end-of-life care issues.

Living wills are most helpful when they identify a *proxy,* an individual who has been authorized to make health care decisions for the impaired elder. A *durable power of attorney* (a legal document) is also helpful. It empowers a competent individual to make health care decisions for an incompetent individual.

Family members are not without support. Medical professionals are also closely involved in end-of-life medical decision-making. These professionals can help family members weigh the benefits and burdens of treatments. They can provide information about the likely outcomes of specific choices and options. And they can help the family chart a course.

Uncertainty (difficulty in knowing) and ambivalence (difficulty in deciding) surround end-of-life decisions. Family members can find themselves disagreeing with one another—a common and natural part of the end-of-life experience. And they can also find themselves disagreeing with individuals outside the family—with friends and associates (even medical professionals) who question or challenge family decisions.

Thus, once again, the family must find ways to operate

as a cohesive team—sharing feelings and participating in the decision-making process. They must be comfortable with their decisions. And this comfort, we think, derives from the knowledge that decisions have been guided by the family's values, the wishes of the elder, and the best interests of the family.

Family input into end-of-life decision-making is critical. Family members possess both a right and a responsibility to participate in end-of-life decision-making. This involvement helps ensure a "good death" for the elder—one that focuses on comfort and dignity within the context of a caring environment.

Close involvement in the elder's "dying well process" helps ease the elder's suffering. It helps family members accept the reality of imminent death, and it enables the family to make its final goodbyes.

Task two: say goodbye to the illness

The Alzheimer's journey can seem interminable. The progressive nature of the illness—its relentless care demands—can eventually dominate family life. And the family can find itself engulfed by the illness—consumed by the mounting care demands and challenged by the increasing emotional and psychological stresses.

Family members, who have been saying "goodbye" to the elder throughout the Alzheimer's journey, now, toward the end, see a time when they can also say goodbye to the illness.

Yet, many family members find it difficult to "let go" of the illness—to finally say "goodbye" and to begin imagin-

ing life without the illness. The family can find itself cling-
ing to the illness—holding on and neglecting the need to reorganize and reinvest in family life.

Thus, family members, in Phase Seven, face the task of
"letting go"—of expelling the "invader" (the illness) from
family life and reclaiming family life. This "letting go" process occurs in steps—over time. And it involves a change in
family identity. It involves a moving *away* from the sense
that "we are an Alzheimer's family"—and *toward* the sense
that "we are *no longer* an Alzheimer's family."

The first step in this process is to recognize the *void*—
the empty space in family life that the end of the illness has
left behind. Family members feel the void—the loss of a
role. Certain family members may, for example, have developed excellent caregiving skills—and a caregiving role—
that are no longer useful. They may have developed close
relationships with health care professionals—and with
other Alzheimer's families—that are now languishing.

Thus, family members, in Phase Seven, face the challenge of adapting not only to the loss of the elder but also to
the "loss" of the illness—and to the loss of a caregiving role
and a set of relationships.

The second step in the "letting go" process is to reflect
on the Alzheimer's journey, to look back on its course and
to consider its effect on family life. This reflection can help
family members gain perspective on the Alzheimer's experience. It can help them see their accomplishments and
understand their triumphs—the challenges they've faced
and overcome. And it can help them see the Alzheimer's experience in its *entirety*—a necessary step in understanding
the significance of the family's efforts and achievements.

Families can (and should) take pride in their care contributions—in the ways they've contributed to their loved one's safety, comfort, dignity, and quality of life. Yet, many family members reach the end with a sense that their efforts have been inadequate and futile—that it's all been for naught. Feelings of guilt and regret can linger. And ongoing pain and sadness can interfere with the family's need to reorganize and move forward.

Dialogue between and among family members can help relieve feelings of guilt and regret. Dialogue and reflection can help family members recognize and appreciate their care efforts—and can help them "let go" of the illness.

Family members might consider the ways in which the family has *benefited* from the Alzheimer's experience. The disease has imposed burdens on family life. But it has provided opportunities for personal growth—and it may have strengthened family bonds.

Family members will find it useful, in Phase Seven, to consider what they've learned—about family life and about one another. They will find it useful to reflect on the transformed family boundary, structure, and culture.

How have our roles, relationships, and expectations changed? How do we now define and prioritize our values? How have we grown and adapted? What do we take with us into the future? What should we leave behind? Answers to these questions (and others) will help family members appreciate their experience—and will help the family move more effectively toward closure.

Moreover, reflection and dialogue will help family members understand the nature of the Alzheimer's journey—its meaning and significance. These meanings are constructed (in part at least) through family conversations that seek to "make sense" of the illness—that seek to construct a "story" about the family's experience.

This story (and the telling of the story) helps family members gain closure with both the elder *and* the illness. It helps them "let go" of the illness. And it helps them recognize that the family has truly reached the end of the Alzheimer's journey.

The family journey will continue. And one major step in the Phase Seven adaptation process is the reclaiming of family life—which begins with the process of "reclaiming" the elder.

Task three: honor the legacy

In addition to "letting go" of the illness, family members, in Phase Seven, must begin the process of "reclaiming" the elder, of regaining a memory of the individual they once knew—before the illness.

This process requires some effort. Family members tend to retain the last picture of the elder—a picture of a frail, confused, dependent, incompetent individual struggling to maintain some measure of human dignity. The family tends to retain a vivid memory of this picture—and a less vivid memory of the strong, capable individual they once knew.

The lingering memory of the impaired elder can crowd out memories of the non-impaired elder—the "whole" individual who once occupied such a unique and important place in family life. But through stories and recollections, family members can begin to recover the memory of the loved on they once knew—before illness exacted its toll.

Through reclaiming the whole person—through recalling a picture of the "whole" individual—family members can retain the loved one's psychological and emotional presence in family life. And they can move forward with a legacy that will remain alive for generations.

The "reclaiming process," as we noted, occurs through conversations about the elder—through recollections of special experiences and events. By telling stories, reviewing old pictures and photographs, examining familiar and favorite objects, and recalling memorable times, family members can keep the loved one "alive." They can maintain his or her psychological presence in family life, and they can move forward with the legacy.

Individual family members can engage in this reclaiming process—"on their own" (individually), but the experience is far more meaningful and powerful when family members make it a shared family activity—a shared experience that helps the family find meaning and closure.

Task four: reclaim family life

Throughout the Alzheimer's journey, the family has increasingly found itself organizing around the illness—and increasingly surrendering certain parts of family life. With the end of the journey, family members must consciously begin to reclaim family life. They must "let go" of the illness and begin "filling the void." And the first step in filling this void is to reinvest in family life and relationships—to reorganize and take up familiar activities and routines.

During the course of the illness, family members, in Phase Seven, have necessarily focused on short-term perspectives and here-and-now concerns. And they may have lost sight of the long view. They may have lost (temporarily) the ability to focus on their own hopes and aspirations—and enjoyments.

Thus family members, in Phase Seven, must find ways to renew interest in recreational activities and hobbies—pursuits that may have been crowded out by the illness. They must look for ways to reengage with one another—to strengthen communications and to share enjoyments. They must find ways to reinvest in the family's vision. And they renew and maintain the family *activities* and *relationships* that support that vision.

This reinvestment in aspirations, relationships, and enjoyments can point the family toward the future—while retaining connections to the past. It can help family members retain the positive elements of their experience—while leaving behind the rest.

The Alzheimer's journey comes finally and inevitably to an end. But the family journey continues—a journey that carries with it the memory of perseverance, courage, and faith in the face of dementing illness.

CHAPTER TWELVE

Understanding Behavior Problems

Introduction

IN THE PRECEDING CHAPTERS (CHAPTERS FIVE THROUGH eleven), we described the issues surrounding each phase of the Alzheimer's journey, and we laid out the tasks for addressing those issues. We've not thus far addressed the behavior problems associated with Alzheimer's disease, since they can occur at any point in the illness—they're not tied directly to any specific phase.

Nonetheless, these behavior problems remain the most pernicious and troubling and baffling parts of the illness. They endanger the elder; they frustrate caregivers; and they hold the potential for exhausting and undermining family life.

But what do we mean by "problem behaviors?" What's their source and nature? Why are they so troubling? And what's their effect on family life?

Behavior problems: definition and source

Problem behaviors can be seen as behaviors that *bother* someone—that bother and trouble the elder, the caregivers, family members, and other community members. These behaviors, often unpredictable in nature, are generally socially unacceptable and difficult to "live with." They disrupt normal family routines, rituals, and relationships. And they disorganize family life.

Behavior problems take various forms:

Delusions
Delusions are beliefs and opinions that are clearly not true—but continue to be strongly held. Afflicted elders may believe, for example, that family members (and others) are stealing their possessions, or plotting against them, or deceiving them (claiming to be other than who they are). These delusions lack any rational basis, but their grip is strong. And attempts to dismiss them (to explain them away) may simply strengthen the elder's belief in them.

Hallucinations
Hallucinations are false or distorted perceptions of objects and events, and they can be both auditory and (more commonly) visual. The elder may see objects floating in space—or hear voices and music. Certain kinds of stimulation can precipitate hallucinations. An elder may see a reflection in a window or mirror— and conclude that he or she is being observed.

The elder may hear certain sounds (the sound of a radio)—and conclude that the house has been invaded. Many hallucinations occur without the influence of outside stimulation.

Agitation

Agitation can take the form of restlessness, jitteriness, and general upset. Agitated individuals may engage in purposeless and repetitive activities. They may, for example, repeatedly pace the floor or repeatedly change articles of clothing. Or they may wander—and become lost.

Aggression

Aggression can take the form of unprovoked verbal and physical attacks. Elders may engage in *reactive* aggression—they may strike out at a caregiver who's providing help or who seems to be invading body space. And they may engage in *predatory* aggression—they may physically attack and attempt to injure another individual. Elders may experience a *catastrophic* reaction—they may abruptly lose emotional control and develop feelings of panic, rage, and despair.

Mood disorders

Mood disorders lead to a range of unhappy feelings. These disorders can express themselves in tearfulness, fearfulness, obsessiveness, expressions of worthlessness, and stated desires to "end it all."

These troubling behaviors and states of mind develop over time, and it's tempting to conclude that they're caused solely by the disease. But their origins are complex. And they're influenced by various factors—by factors within the elder's personality, within the social environment, and within the elder's set of relationships.

Effective approaches to problem behaviors require an understanding of all these factors—and a clear view of the ways in which they all interrelate and interact to produce specific behaviors. And the first step toward more effective approaches is to see the ways in which *behavior problems* differ from *cognitive symptoms.*

Cognitive symptoms, as we noted in Chapter Three, derive from damaged brain structures. And impairment occurs in six general domains:

Memory
Afflicted individuals initially encounter memory difficulties. They grow increasingly absent-minded and forgetful, and they lose ability to learn new material—and to remember previously learned material. In advanced stages, they may lose the ability to identify family members—or even to remember their own names.

Language
Afflicted individuals lose language skills. Initially, they may encounter difficulty in choosing words. In time, they begin to rely on fewer and fewer words. Their conversation becomes increasingly vague and empty. And they even-

tually lose full ability to use written and spoken language.

Praxis

Afflicted individuals lose the ability to plan, initiate, and conduct tasks. They may engage in needless, repetitive activities. And they may lose the
ability to make simple and familiar gestures—
and to use familiar implements and tools.

Visuospatial

Afflicted individuals lose the ability to orient
themselves within their physical environment.
They may wander and become lost. They lose
the ability to fully interpret visual stimuli—to
recognize and identify familiar faces and objects. They may, for example, lose the ability to
correctly draw the face of a clock—and then
place the hands at a specific time.

Judgement and reasoning

Afflicted individuals lose judgment and reasoning skills. They may act impulsively and
take risks (driving risks, for example). They
may make unrealistic assessments of their abilities—and engage in unusual and inappropriate behavior.

Attention and concentration

Afflicted individuals lose the ability to maintain focus and concentration and to sustain
purposeful, long–term activity. They may lose
sight of a task's purpose—or become easily distracted, especially in busy social settings.

These *cognitive impairments* are progressive and irreversible in nature. They come and they stay. Afflicted individuals may have good days and bad days—and even days when they seem almost normal. But cognitive impairments inevitably worsen over time. Memory inevitably fades; judgement falters; and thinking skills steadily decline.

Behavior problems present a different picture, and they differ significantly from *cognitive impairments*. These behavior problems are neither progressive nor irreversible. They may come and go—they don't necessarily come and stay. An elder, for example, may hallucinate for several months—and then stop hallucinating. Moreover, not all dementia patients experience behavior problems, although most will exhibit some kind of troublesome behavior.

Cognitive impairments derive from one source—changes in the brain structure. *Behavior problems*, however, seem to derive from several sources—from several factors operating together. Let's look briefly at some major influences.

Individual factors

Behavior is influenced by factors within the individual—by progressive brain damage and loss in brain function, which impairs overall mental function. Elders find it increasingly difficult to think and remember—and to correctly perceive and interpret the world. These distortions—these changes in perceptions and interpretations—undermine the ability to think clearly and to act appropriately.

Physical and psychological problems can also affect behavior. Nutritional status, medications, infections, pain, and overall physical debilitation can contribute to problem behaviors. Self-esteem and emotional balance issues—together with specific symptoms (depression, for example)—can also lead to troublesome behaviors.

Environment

The elder's physical and social environment can heavily influence behavior. Too much stimulation, for example, can cause agitation—too little can cause boredom. A confusing environment—one that's difficult to interpret—can lead the elder into delusions and hallucinations.

Relationships

The elder's family relationships—the ways in which family members relate and respond—critically influence behavior. Conflicted and emotionally troubled relationships can create turmoil and distress—and can exacerbate existing behavior problems. Escalating problem behaviors can begin to undermine family relationships. And the elder can begin to feel increasingly isolated and alone—vulnerable to even more behavior problems.

All these factors—individual, environmental, and relational—interact and interrelate to produce specific behaviors. And problem behaviors, we believe, must be understood in terms of *all* the factors that influence and shape the elder's actions.

Too often, however, family members focus on one area—on one single influence. And they take the actions they think will relieve a specific problem. Family members may, for example, use medications to change the elder's mood or physical condition. Or they may change the living environment—making it less challenging and less stimulating (or more challenging and more stimulating).

These kinds of responses (linear or cause and effect responses) are understandable, and they often provide relief. But a comprehensive response (a systems approach) to problem behavior requires that family members consider all the factors that might be influencing behavior—including factors in the elder, in the environment, and in the elder's family relationships.

This systems approach recognizes that one factor, operating alone, can (by itself) increase the likelihood that a behavior problem will occur. But several factors operating together—interacting and interrelating (feeding off one another)—can significantly increase the frequency and seriousness of behavior problems.

The behavior issues are complex, and family members often feel overwhelmed by the complexities surrounding behavior problems. ("How can we sort it all out?" "Where do we begin?" "Is there any hope for relieving problems?")

Family members can, we think, address these problems within the context of the family system. And a good beginning point, we think, is to look first at the elder—and attempt to see the world as he or she sees it. Look first at the ways in which cognitive impairments are affecting the elder's *perceptions* and *interpretations* of the world. And then try to see the world from the elder's perspective—from his or her unique set of *perceptions* and *interpretations*.

Perceptions and interpretations

Each human being perceives and interprets the world in his or her unique way. And, although individual perceptions and interpretations differ, members of a similar group (a family, for example) tend to stay generally "in sync" with those around them.

Even when individuals (including family members) hold differing perceptions and interpretations, they're often able to resolve them through communication—through dialogue that resolves differences and fosters shared understandings.

Alzheimer's disease creates a special problem—and a new set of issues. The afflicted elder, steadily losing cognitive abilities (memory, concentration, judgement), is steadily losing the ability to accurately perceive and interpret the world.

For the impaired elder, the world is becoming a different place—it is *diverging* from the world that most of us know and understand. And, in the face of this increasing divergence, family members face a major challenge. They must begin to see and understand the elder's world—from his or her perspective. They must begin to see the world from the "inside out"—through the elder's eyes.

Diverging worlds

The impaired elder—steadily losing a memory of the past, a sense of the present, and a vision of the future—is moving into an increasingly narrow, "here-and-now" world. Family members struggle to understand this world. And they struggle to understand the difficult behaviors that accompany this move into a "new world." They strive to "manage" and "control" difficult behaviors—while striving to maintain emotional and psychological connections with the elder.

These efforts to "manage" behavior are understandable—and commendable. Certain forms of behavior "management" are useful—and often necessary. Medications, for example, can relieve mental and physical symptoms. And changes in the environment—changes, for example, in the level of stimulation (up or down)—can reduce frustration and agitation.

But these efforts to "control" and "manage" behavior often (almost invariably) fail to consider the elder's diverging world. They fail to consider the ways in which the elder's changing perceptions and interpretations are influencing his or her behavior.

Thus, as we noted, the first step in understanding problem behaviors is to begin seeing the world as the elder sees it—distorted as it may seem. And the key to this world—the key to greater understanding—is a human quality called *empathy.*

Empathy

Empathy—the ability to understand and identify with another's circumstances, feelings, and motives—provides a *bridge* into the afflicted elder's world.

Empathy helps family members "bridge into" the

elder's world—and see it from his or her perspective. The exercise of empathy allows family members to begin "working with the elder"—instead of "working on the elder." And it allows family members to begin working from the "inside out"—*to begin the process of matching expectations to the elder's reality.*

Expectations lie at the heart of the family's responses to problem behaviors. Expectations shape the ways in which family members relate to their increasingly impaired loved one. And expectations greatly influence family members' responses to specific behavior problems. Let's look more closely at this critical concept.

Expectations

As we noted, a problem behavior is a behavior that bothers someone—that bothers and troubles the elder, a family member, a friend, a neighbor, or some other community member. These behaviors are bothersome for various reasons—but especially for the ways in which they violate expectations.

But what exactly are expectations? How do they work? How do they affect us? What's their relation to problem behaviors?

Expectations can be seen as a set of beliefs, convictions, and opinions about what an individual *can* do—and *ought* to do. These expectations shape our interactions and interrelations with others. And they shape our responses to unanticipated behaviors—to the unexpected behavior, for example, of an impaired elder.

We're disturbed by behavior that fails to meet established expectations, and we often react strongly. But why are we so disturbed? What troubles us? What's the source of our strong reactions?

Reactions to unpredictable behavior are shaped by both our *experience* and our *values*.

Experience

Our expectations for others rests heavily on our experience—on the nature of our interactions and interrelations with those around us. Over time, we develop beliefs about how others will behave. We construct expectations. And we come to believe that friends, family members, and others will meet those expectations—most of the time. We count on it.

Some of these expectations remain fluid and dynamic. We expect children to change, for example, and we assume that we will change our expectations for them—as they grow and develop. Most expectations, however, eventually become stable and predictable. We come to expect that friends and family members will act in predictable ways. And we're surprised (often upset) by unexpected behavior—by behavior that fails to meet our established expectations.

Demented elders pose special problems. Their cognitive impairments distort their perceptions and interpretations—and affect their ability to maintain a consistent and predictable pattern of behavior.

These unpredictable behaviors create a gap between the *is* and the *ought*—between the reality (the behavior that's occurring) and the expectations (the behavior that family members think ought to occur).

Family members feel this gap—this difference between reality and expectations. They feel the tension and frustration surrounding unmet expectations. And they seek answers to difficult questions. What's the cause of our elder's behavior? Why is it so bothersome? How should we respond? Why are we reacting so strongly?

Values

Our expectations rest also on a foundation of *values*—on our "conceptions of the desirable." We rank these values. We place them in a "values hierarchy," and we rank them according the importance we attach to each. These values shape our specific behaviors and goals. ("What's important?" "What's less important?") And we hold closely to them. We strive to maintain the established value hierarchy—we're reluctant to reorder it.

We expect family members and friends (and others) to establish appropriate goals and to conduct themselves in appropriate ways. And we're disturbed when a loved one's behavior violates strongly-held values—when it violates a social norm, for example, or transgresses a well-established "rule."

Moreover, we're often surprised by our strong reactions to unanticipated and unwanted behaviors. ("It angers me when Dad interrupts conversations? Why can't he exercise some simple courtesy?")

These strong emotional reactions are understandable. Unwanted and undesirable behaviors violate certain closely-held personal and family values. We react strongly to these "values violations"—even when we understand that they are rooted in cognitive impairments and dementia-related disorders.

Alzheimer's family members face especially difficult values issues. Although the fundamental family values may stay intact, individual family members face ongoing values challenges—they must constantly reorder values in ways that recognize losses and take into account new realities. ("It's alright if Dad dresses in old clothes—it doesn't really matter." "I expect that Mom will interrupt at times—and won't always act in socially appropriate ways. But, after all, courtesy isn't the highest value at this point.")

Acceptance of the elder requires some reordering of the value hierarchy—some change in the way family members rank certain values. Acceptance requires a change in the priority one attaches to a specific value. This ability to reprioritize values—the first step in a "new" approach to problem behaviors—can lead to changed responses. And changed responses can lead to changed behaviors. Acceptance (of both the elder *and* his or her unpredictable behaviors) can reduce frustration and ease the family's sense of fatalism—the sense that no action or response will ultimately change *anything*.

All families experience frustration—but the Alzheimer's family experiences special frustrations. This sense of frustration and futility is compounded by an inability to effectively communicate with the elder—to negotiate expectations and to address problems in usual ways.

This inability to effectively communicate reminds family members of their elder's progressive and irreversible losses. The "communication breakdown" daily reminds family members that they are dealing with a changed (and changing) loved one—a reality that evokes feelings of grief and sadness.

Finally, impaired elders simply don't understand their circumstances. They don't understand their declining ability to make sound judgments and to exercise old skills and abilities. And, consequently, they're unable to establish and meet realistic expectations for *themselves.*

Many family members—coping daily with increasingly bothersome problem behaviors—continue to rely on various forms of control and restraint (medications, behavioral management techniques). They continue to "force" certain behaviors—to impel behaviors that are more socially acceptable and easier "to live with."

These attempts to "force" changes in behavior, however, usually fall short. And they lead often to undesirable and unintended consequences. In the face of failed attempts to change behavior, family members can find themselves stepping back from one another—emotionally distancing themselves from the elder and from one another. Over time, frustration can build; relationships can deteriorate; and behavior problems can steadily worsen.

Toward a new approach

Behavior problems, as we noted, derive from several sources—they're influenced by several factors. And no single approach can finally eliminate or, perhaps, even relieve a problem.

We are suggesting an approach, however, that we believe can help family members relieve frustration and turmoil—and find more effective ways for "working with" the elder. This approach is based on our clinical experience and our direct work with Alzheimer's families.

The approach asks family members first to accept the elder—with all his or her impairments and behavior problems. Through acceptance, family members can begin to see the world through the elder's eyes—the first step in adjusting expectations. They can then begin the process of matching expectations to reality—of "working with the elder" rather than "on the elder."

Let's look more closely at the process for examining, understanding, and revising expectations.

Steps toward a new approach

Step one: match expectations to capabilities

Expectations shape perceptions and interpretations—and they color family members' assessments of the elder's capabilities. Thus, family members, in their new approach, must first examine their expectations—they must ask themselves what they *think* the elder *can* do. ("What can we reasonably expect?" "Which expectations must we now examine?" "Which ones must we change?")

Realistic expectations change the way behavior is perceived. And they help relieve feelings of frustration—and even anger. An elder's refusal to comply with a routine request, for example, can seem like a form of stubbornness—when, in fact, the elder may simply be unable to meet an expectation. He or she may simply be unable to carry out a specific task (dressing appropriately, for example, or socializing in an acceptable manner).

Expectations, as we noted, shape our perceptions and interpretations, and they influence our responses to events and behaviors. When family members change their expectations for their elder, they change the ways in which they respond to difficult behaviors. When they change their responses, they increase their opportunities for changing unwanted behaviors.

Moreover, when family members change expectations—when they bring them into line with the elder's capabilities—they reduce emotional "distancing." They maintain a stronger emotional connection to the elder, and they enhance their ability to maintain a stronger relationship.

In our experience, appropriate and realistic expectations, make behaviors seem less troublesome. They reduce the gap between the *is* and the *ought*. And they reduce frustration and tension—for both the elder and his or her family members.

Step two: match expectations to values and goals

After asking themselves what the elder *can* do, family members must then ask themselves what the elder *should* do. Family members must reflect on their values and goals. ("What's important?" "What's not important?")

They then must begin to reprioritize their values and goals in ways that match new understandings of the elder's capabilities. With new understandings about what the elder *can* do—and a reordering of values—family members can then begin to develop new expectations about what the elder *should* do.

Step three: bridge into the elder's world

Realistic assessments of the elder's capabilities, can help family members "bridge" into the elder's world—a first step in addressing important questions. (What perceptions and interpretations are guiding our elder's behavior? How can we understand behaviors from the elder's perspective? Given our new understandings and perspectives, how does the elder's behavior "make sense?")

Step four: explore new approaches for addressing undesirable behaviors

With a view of the elder's world—from the elder's perspective—family members can then begin to adjust their expectations. In so doing, they will find themselves reacting in new ways—and discovering new ways of "working with" the elder. They will find ways to preserve their relationship with the elder—while maintaining a calmer and more peaceful environment.

Changing expectations: a family task

All these steps can help *individual* family members develop fresh approaches to problem behaviors. But, as we've noted throughout the book, the family achieves greater success when it works together—when it uses dialogue to examine issues and to formulate courses of action. This team approach provides some specific benefits—for some specific reasons.

First, when all family members work together, they find ways to support one another—while facing up to revised expectations that create pain and sadness. This team approach can lead to greater consensus—and to more effective care approaches.

Second, a team approach, supported by family dialogue, helps family members identify expectations that cause tension—or that are not fully understood. A team approach allows family members to share their knowledge of the elder—and to jointly develop new expectations.

Finally, as family members change their expectations for the elder, they will necessarily need to change expectations for themselves—and they will need to discuss these new expectations. A team approach (supported by family dialogue) allows all family members to express their concerns—and to share their feelings about changed and changing expectations.

Conclusion

Expectations, as we noted, influence perceptions of the elder and interpretations of his or her behavior. By changing expectations, family members close the gap between the *is* and the *ought*. They bring their expectations into congruence with the elder's capabilities. And they change their emotional responses to problem behaviors—thereby increasing the potential for changing unwanted behaviors.

This approach may seem to some like a form of "surrender"—a kind of "giving up" to problem behaviors. And it may seem (to some) like meager advice—a futile set of coping efforts that holds little potential for changing *any* kind of behavior.

Our experience tells us, however, that the ability to

change expectations holds out opportunities for "working with" the elder—and for relieving tension, frustration, and emotional conflict. The ability to change expectations can lead to changed responses—and to changed behaviors in the elder.

Our family system perspective is intended to provide additional tools for addressing difficult behavior problems. Yet, despite the family's best efforts, undesirable behaviors often persist—and they can slowly (or dramatically) escalate.

In the face of ongoing and progressively difficult problem behaviors, family members should seek the kinds of help that physicians and other health care professionals provide. These professionals can help family members develop approaches to undesirable behaviors, and they can support the family as it formulates and tests new approaches.

Moreover, medical professionals can often prescribe psychotropic drugs that relieve specific problems. Medications can, for example, relieve hallucinations and delusions. Antidepressants can relieve gloom and depression.

We urge family members to work closely with physicians and other health professionals who deal directly with dementia-related behavior problems. These professionals can provide an entry point into the array of community services—and they can provide invaluable ongoing support and guidance.

CHAPTER THIRTEEN

Teaching Stories

Introduction

THROUGHOUT THE BOOK, WE HAVE SHARED VARIOUS ideas about family life—and about the Alzheimer's journey. Behind these ideas lie stories—dramatic tales of courage, perseverance, and ingenuity in the face of dementing illness. In this chapter, we have gathered together some "teaching stories"—accounts of the ways in which families have developed unique approaches to their unique care problems.

These "teaching stories" have been used in many fields, including philosophy, psychology, and the humanities. They are similar to fables—except that they don't offer a moral point. Instead, they're intended to illuminate new ideas, to clarify concepts, and to show the complexities surrounding various issues.

The stories in this chapter are drawn from our clinical practice experience. The facts are real—the families are fictitious. The events we describe have been drawn from the experiences of various families—and then pulled into one short story. This method allows us to guard the privacy of specific families—while presenting "real life" experiences.

We hope these teaching stories will help family members step back and see new options—new opportunities for addressing care challenges. We think that close rereading of the stories will generate new insights and illuminate fresh approaches to difficult Alzheimer's care issues. We hope family members will read the stories together—and discuss them. Family members might wish to discuss and analyze their own stories—and draw insights from their own family discussions.

Mr. B.

Mr. B.'s wife had been struggling with Alzheimer's disease for about five years, and she was becoming increasingly aggressive. She needed help in almost all areas and had recently begun to wet and soil herself.

Mr. B.'s physician recommended that he take Mrs. B. to the bathroom every two hours. But the trips were becoming nightmarish. Mrs. B. would initially refuse requests to use the toilet. But with some coaxing and pleading she would relent, and Mr. B. would escort her into the bathroom. Once there, she would sit appropriately on the toilet—but would refuse to take down her pants. When Mr. B. would attempt to take them down, Mrs. B. would strike out at him—hitting and scratching and shouting obscenities.

In consultations with a family therapist, Mr. B. first defined his expectations. He expected that his wife would understand the need to use the toilet and would comprehend and follow his directions. But Mrs. B's illness had progressed, and she was unable to comprehend instructions—even though she gave the impression that she understood spoken language.

Mr. B. was advised to "bridge" into Mrs. B's world—and to see it from her perspective. Given Mrs. B's inability to understand her toileting needs and to comprehend instructions, her husband's requests were meaningless. Moreover, the act of taking down her pants represented a highly unwanted intrusion—even an assault.

By letting go of established expectations—by seeing the world through his wife's eyes—Mr. B. was able to formulate a new approach. He knew that Mrs. B. enjoyed looking at pictures of their grandchildren. So he hung pictures of the grandchildren along the hallway leading to the bathroom. Instead of asking Mrs. B. to visit the bathroom, Mr. B. began asking her to view the pictures, which she would do—one by one down the length of the hallway.

When they reached the bathroom, Mrs. B. seemed to understand her need to use the toilet. But then Mr. B. faced the task of taking down the pants. Again, Mr. B. bridged into his wife's world—and was able to understand his wife's embarrassment. He covered his wife with a large towel, and, with the towel in place, he was able to lower her pants and successfully toilet her.

Sarah C.

Sarah C. faced an increasingly perplexing behavior problem. Her mother, living in an assisted living facility, had begun to imagine that her elderly next-door neighbors were slipping under her door at night and stealing her possessions. When Sarah's mother could not find a belonging, she would angrily confront the couple—and make angry accusations. She had also begun to complain regularly to the facility's management. Sarah's attempts to reason with her mother—to talk her out of the delusion—only evoked more anger and frustration.

Knowing that her mother was a very religious person, Sarah suggested that she begin praying for her neighbors. This activity seemed to relieve Mrs. C's anger and fear, and Sarah was able to discuss the apartment arrangements. Through discussion, Sarah and her mother were able to find a "safer" place to live. Mrs. C. moved into a nursing home that contained a special care unit for Alzheimer's patients—and she made a good adjustment.

Mr. D.

Mr. D. enjoyed taking his wife to dinner, but the restaurant experience invariably became unpleasant. At some point, Mrs. D. would become angry and agitated, and Mr. D. would have to take her back home—sometimes before even being seated.

In consultation with a therapist, Mr. D. was asked to provide a detailed account of the restaurant trips, and he related this experience. On the way to the restaurant, Mrs. D. would remain calm and composed. If they were not immediately seated, however, Mrs. D. would become tense and impatient—and she would sometimes noisily express her anger.

Once seated, Mr. D. would allow his wife to peruse the menu—hoping that she would comprehend it. Often Mrs. D. would simply stare at the menu until Mr. D. either assisted her—or placed the order himself. While waiting for the dinner, Mrs. D. would often become angry—and would begin shouting and gesticulating.

During the consultation, Mr. D. acknowledged that his expectations for his wife were unrealistic. Waiting for a table irritated her. Attempting to read a menu frustrated her. And waiting for the dinner upset her.

Mr. D. formulated a new approach. He began to make reservations at times when he and Mrs. D. could be immediately seated. He informed the waitress that they didn't need a menu—he could place the orders. And he asked the waitress to immediately bring a salad or a cup of soup—a dining activity that occupied them while they waited for the main course.

Molly J.

Molly paid a visit to her mother—and found her hiding in fear behind the curtains. Mom stated that she could see a group of men outside the house—staring at her and preparing to invade her domain. Molly understood the futility of reasoning with her mother—and attempting to talk her out of the delusion. Instead she said, "Those poor men. They should be home with their families. Let's go to the kitchen and make some cookies for them." While making the cookies, Molly and her mother chatted and relaxed. When the cookies were finally made, the men had "disappeared"—Molly had entirely forgotten about them.

Joe and Betty

Joe's dementia had been worsening, and Betty's care duties were becoming increasingly burdensome. Betty informed their eight children (all of whom lived nearby) that it would be a great help to have Saturdays off—free from care duties. Each child agreed to donate one Saturday every other month—a seemingly workable plan.

The arrangement, however, soon broke down. The children were not prepared to meet the care challenges. On the first Saturday, the youngest daughter returned her father, stating that she could not manage him *and* care for her preschool children.

The children met and developed a different approach. They decided to work in groups of two and three. And they set up a series of activities that would occupy their father—without unduly frustrating and taxing the caregivers (the children). The children then agreed to meet once a month to review and discuss the arrangements.

Rudy

Rudy, a successful businessman, had suffered a series of strokes that impaired his ability to speak and to comprehend language. His daughter, Judy, a lawyer, had been granted power of attorney (by both parents) to deal with various property and financial issues. Judy, however, seemed unable to take the necessary steps. Although she understood her responsibilities, she seemed unable to act.

In a family conference, family members noted that Rudy had always made the family decisions. He had always been fully "in charge." And family members had come to trust his leadership and judgement—they relied on it and deferred to it. Upon reflection, Judy began to see that her decision-making difficulties derived from her instinctive need to seek her father's approval. She was reluctant to act without Rudy's final OK—but it was an OK that Rudy could no longer provide.

Judy began working on family matters in Rudy's presence. In his presence, she found herself addressing family business and financial matters confidently and effectively. Her father's presence gave her the "permission" she needed to proceed.

Joan

Joan's mother had grown increasingly confused, and she had begun telephoning Joan repeatedly. The calls would begin around 8:00 A.M. and would continue throughout the day—coming in sometimes eight to ten times per hour. Joan's mother usually could not explain why she was calling, and she would often ask the same question over and over—throughout the day. She did not, however, call any of Joan's three siblings—for a reason. She used the telephone's speed dialer, and Joan's number was in the first position. She would dial Joan's number, but she would not go to any of the other numbers.

In a family conference, Joan and her siblings formulated an approach to their Mother's behavior problem. First, they agreed to take turns occupying the first position on the speed dialer—and share the responsibility for fielding Mom's calls. This strategy eased some of Joan's stress, but it did not stop the phone calls.

The family members then concluded that the phone calls were an expression of their mother's anxiety. So they began calling her throughout the day—beginning early before she had an opportunity to initiate her own calls. This strategy seemed to reassure Mom that her children were thinking about her—and that she was not alone. The children were able to make the calls on their own schedule and reduce the number of Mom's calls.

Martha

Martha's dementia had worsened, and she could no longer live safely at home. But she refused to consider an assisted living center—stating that she had built the home with her husband and wanted to die there.

The community, however, lacked the kind of care services that could maintain Martha in her home—home care was not an option. Martha badly needed another living arrangement. But when her daughter and son-in-law attempted to discuss a move to a facility, Martha would become angry and tearful. Her family members did not wish to force Martha from her home, but they feared for her safety.

In a family meeting, family members recalled that Martha enjoyed family get-togethers—especially those that involved her grandchildren. They decided to hold a series of family get-togethers and visit some facilities together—as a family. Martha was not asked to choose a facility, and the visits were followed by an enjoyable family dinner—a positive ending to the day.

During the visits, Martha's grandchildren would talk about grandma's new home—and point out the things they liked about each facility. Martha and the grandchildren especially liked a facility that contained a large collection of birds.

The family concluded that this facility was a good "fit." And they began asking Martha *when* she would like to make the move—they moved the conversation away from *whether* to *when*. Martha decided that she would like to enjoy one last Christmas at home. The family celebrated Christmas together at home—and then celebrated New Year's day together in the care facility. Martha had accepted the move, and the family's concern about her safety and well-being had eased.

Phil

Phil's dementia had worsened, and he could no longer walk or talk. He spent most of his days in a semi-conscious state, and he had begun to choke and gag on his food. A softer diet did not relieve the choking problem, and Phil began to lose weight.

The nursing home summoned Phil's physician, and the physician scheduled a family meeting to discuss treatment options—which included the use of a feeding tube. Phil had not completed a living will, and the family was unsure about how to proceed.

The physician asked Phil's family members to reflect on the family history and to recall the family's experience with death and dying. They recalled the death of Phil's mother, and they recalled how disturbed Phil had been by the sight of feeding tubes and wrist restraints. He stated at the time that he wished to avoid such an experience.

These recollections helped Phil's family members reach their decision. They decided to try a feeding tube. But Phil became agitated and tried to remove the tube. The nurse then suggested the use of wrist restraints. The family knew that Phil would not approve this procedure, and they asked the nurse to remove the feeding tube. Phil's weight declined and he developed pneumonia—an illness that ended his life. His family members were with him when he died.

Jerry

As Jerry's dementia worsened, his family members found themselves struggling to meet increasing care demands. Moreover, they found themselves increasingly in conflict with one another. Over the years, arguments and misunderstandings had undermined family relationships. And conflict and turmoil continually disrupted the family care strategy meetings.

Jerry's son-in-law, a computer expert, proposed an innovative solution. He constructed a family web site—a place where family members could exchange messages and discuss care problems and issues. Freed from the need to hold face-to-face meetings, the family members developed an effective team approach to Jerry's care. They developed successful care approaches. Long-standing hurts and angers faded, and a new sense of connection emerged.

Conclusion

These teaching stories illustrate the kinds of creative care approaches that family members can achieve when they work together—as a team. Although the Alzheimer's journey is fraught with dangers and challenges, millions of American families find ways to cope with the illness—while maintaining family cohesion and well-being. We hope these stories will provide a vision, and we hope they will help family members construct their own unique approaches to their own unique care challenges.

Suggested Readings

Boss, Pauline. *Ambiguous Loss: Learning to Live With Unresolved Grief.* Cambridge: Harvard University Press, 1999. This groundbreaking book details the nature of ambiguous loss and discusses ways in which families can effectively cope with that experience. The book contains an extensive discussion of ambiguous loss as it relates to Alzheimer's disease—and as it affects families who are dealing with an Alzheimer's patient who stays physically present but grows increasingly psychologically absent.

Feil, Naomi. *Validation Breakthrough: Simple Techniques for Communicating with People with Alzheimer's-Type Dementia.* Baltimore: Health Professions Press, 1994. The validation method helps family members address difficult Alzheimer's issues—especially communications issues. This book provides practical advice for relating to Alzheimer's patients—and for maintaining a relationship with them.

Mace, Nancy, Peter Rabins, and Paul McHugh. *The 36-Hour Day: A Guide to Caring for Persons with Alzheimer's*

Disease, Related Dementing Illnesses, and Memory Loss in Later Life. New York: Warner Books, 1992. This classic work has served Alzheimer's families for several decades. It remains essential reading for Alzheimer's family caregivers—and for all others associated with the illness.

McDaniel, Susan (editor), Jeri Hepworth (editor), and William Doherty (editor). *The Shared Experience of Illness: Stories of Patients, Families, and Their Therapists*. New York: Basic Books, 1997. This thirty-four chapter book contains clinicians' accounts of their experiences with families who have coped (or are coping) with chronic illnesses. The book contains a section by Wayne A. Caron, Ph.D., that describes his first experience in leading a support group for Alzheimer's patients.

Pattee, James, M.D., and Orlo Otteson. *The Health Care Future: Defining the Argument, Healing the Debate*. Minneapolis: North Ridge Press, 1997. This book contains a chapter on the nature and function of values and a brief introduction to systems thinking.

Pattee, James, M.D., and Orlo Otteson. *Medical Direction in the Nursing Home: Principles and Concepts for Physician Administrators*. Minneapolis: North Ridge Press, 1991. This book contains a chapter on the role of families in the care of institutionalized elderly. The chapter also provides a brief introduction to some core family system concepts.

Rabins, Peter, Constantine Lyketsos, and Cynthia Steele. *Practical Dementia Care*. New York: Oxford University Press, 1999. This book is aimed at the health care provider.

It describes the nature of dementia, the nature of a diagnosis, and the nature of medical professionals' responses to disease challenges.

Reisberg, Barry. *A Guide to Alzheimer's Disease: For Families, Spouses and Friends.* New York: Free Press, 1983; London: Collier Macmillan, 1981. This book includes the author's model for the Stages of Alzheimer's Disease. As noted in Chapter 3, this information provides an especially good "road map" to the afflicted loved one's journey through the disease stages.

Rolland, John. *Families, Illness, and Disability: An Integrative Treatment Model.* New York: Basic Books, 1994. This pioneering work describes the ways in which illness affects family life—and the ways in which family dynamics evolve over the course of an illness. It provides guidelines for family therapists and other helping professionals.

Steinglass, Peter, Linda Bennett, Steven Wolin, and David Reiss. *The Alcoholic Family.* New York: Basic Books, 1993. This classic text provides an in-depth discussion of family system dynamics. And it discusses some ways in which families can cope with a chronic condition that affects these family dynamics.

Wheatley, Margaret. *Leadership and the New Science.* San Francisco: Berret-Koehler Publishers, 1997. The author, an organizational specialist, provides challenging and cutting-edge views of change, leadership, and the structure of groups.